THE THERAPEUTIC USES OF WRITING

THE

THERAPEUTIC

USES OF

WRITING

Allan Hunter

NOVA SCIENCE PUBLISHERS, INC.

Art Director: Maria Ester Hawrys
Assistant Director: Elenor Kallberg
Graphics: Kerri Pfister, Susan A. Boriotti and
          Frank Grucci
Manuscript Coordinator: Phylis Gaynor
Book Production: Tammy Sauter, Gavin Aghamore,
          Joanne Bennette and Christine Mathosian
Circulation: Gathy De Gregory and Annette Hellinger

Library of Congress Cataloging–in–Publication Data
available upon request

ISBN 1-56072-379-3

© *1996 Nova Science Publishers, Inc.*
  6080 Jericho Turnpike, Suite 207
  Commack, New York 11725
  Tele. 516-499-3103 Fax 516-499-3146
  E Mail Novasci1@aol.com

Printed in the United States of America

TABLE OF CONTENTS

ACKNOWLEDGEMENTS

My debts are far reaching and very varied, but I'll attempt to cover them here. My first debt is to the Peper Harow Foundation, and in particular to David Whitley, who first started me on this way of thinking. To Curry College I owe a debt of gratitude for the chance to teach a series of experimental courses over the years, and in many different settings. Without the support of Dean Fedo, former Dean Keys and the faculty at the Program for the Advancement of Learning, none of this might ever have had a chance to see the light of day. The Dean's fund made money available for the typing of the manuscript, and a sabbatical provided the time necessary to complete the task. Wynne Smith's genius at reading my handwriting was heaven-sent. She had the dubious privilege of seeing all my manuscripts in their first draft, and yet she still remained calm. Maryanne Gallant helped with the transfer of the illustrations and tables to disk, and Marna Maclean completed the task with a patience and graciousness I could only admire. Others who were encouraging when I needed it most include Dr. Ronald Warners, ever tactful and good humored, and Dr. Janice Wagner.

Permission to reproduce the illustrations was most kindly given by a variety of agencies and individuals. For the illustrations in chapter 15 thanks go to Ted Lavash for the two photographs; the four oil paintings by Fayalene Decker Goodman - two of the Dogwood Festival, Greenfield Hill, Ct. ; one untitled; and a street scene, Avallon, France - appear by kind permission of her daughter, Joan Goodman. The four pages of drawings also in chapter 15 came from the archives of Dr. George K. Pratt, by kind permission of his grandaughter, Dr. Susan B. Pratt. W.W. Norton and Co. allowed me to reproduce the diagram by Erik Erikson that appears in chapter 12, and the poetry quoted in chapter 10 is from *Psychopoetry* by Gilbert A. Schloss, copyright © 1976 by Gilbert A. Schloss. It is reprinted here by permission of Grosset and Dunlap, Inc.

All other debts I have attempted to list within the text itself. Some of the games and exercises have been around for a long time, and I do not know where they first originated. I am confident that my own adaptations over the years have made them idiosyncratically 'mine' - if anyone can make such a claim - so if you recognize any of them, do not be alarmed. Certainly Kenneth Koch's excellent *Wishes, Lies, and Dreams* uses the 'I used to...' and 'I seem to be...' games, although I feel our purposes are sufficiently different that I am not intruding on his territory. To the unknown originators of the other games, and the sources that inspired me to make up my own, I owe a debt of gratitude, all the same!

And this brings me to my greatest debt of all - to my students, who took these ideas, developed them, switched them around, made me think, and kept me on my toes at all times. I know that some of you, at least, are still using these ideas and the insights they generated, and I wish you well wherever you are.

The last acknowledgement is a personal one, to Cathy Bennett, and to Anna and Nick Portnoy, and runs deeper than words.

CHAPTER ONE

Statistics tell us, in that heartless way they have, that at the present time approximately half of all marriages in the U.S. end in divorce. As you read this, think how that impacts you. Possibly you have already been through your own divorce or watched your parents do so, or your children. The same statistics inform us that approximately one in three adults will seek psychological counseling for personal distress, and that one in eight will spend time in residential hospitals or homes. Wherever you are, look around. If you are in a public building, a school or library, just try and imagine every eighth person in a psychiatric ward. How many people live in your building? How many are in your family? Which one of your friends is going to suffer? It's pretty sobering.

On the other side of the discussion is the fact that the U.S. currently has just over a million citizens in prison, and another four million under "Correctional Supervision" - which translates as probation, community service, and similar programs. The prison population is going up, and the rehabilitation programs are being cut, so most of these convicts will emerge (and 97% of them *do* hit the streets again) largely unchanged. Or, at least, unchanged for the better. Recidivism - the rate at which convicts are reincarcerated - seems to run at close to 70%. One could conclude that our society, the envy of the free world, is extremely successful at producing criminals and mental distress. Certainly we produce more of them than people with doctoral degrees.

And that is why you need this book. This one, yes, and others like it, too. We are living in very stressful times and my aim is to share with you tactics that can help in preserving your sanity. Now please don't read that as a guarantee. There can be no guarantees here simply because it is not up to me to keep you sane. It is up to you. With the help of these pages, however, I can tell you that you can begin a process that will certainly lead to a better understanding of yourself. Consider this a handbook for dealing with the problems and challenges the world will hurl at you, the sorts of things that might otherwise throw you hopelessly off balance.

Let me give you an example: about fifteen years ago, a friend was hospitalized after attempting to kill herself. When I spoke with her I asked her what the doctors had said. She replied that they had diagnosed her as manic-depressive with paranoid tendencies. She and I talked for a while and then she said to me, "But what does that *mean*, manic-depressive?" The label was nothing that made sense to her. It didn't make sense to me, either. Not surprisingly, it didn't help her to deal with the pain she was going through.

It was thinking about this incident that led me to one of the central thoughts that makes me write this. The doctors, in their wisdom, had labeled her in a way which made sense to them, but not to her. The only problem was that it was her mental distress that needed calming, not theirs. My own thought on this matter is that it does not really matter if the men with initials after their names can give a diagnosis. What has to happen is that the patient has to have a language that allows him or her to understand his or her own distress, in order to move through it. The locus of understanding needs to be returned to the patient.

Another example may clarify this. I was speaking with a student one day at the Liberal Arts college at which I work, and he confided to me that three years of therapy had not helped. "It never did anything for me," he grumbled. I was hardly surprised, since the very words he used suggested that he should be passive, that everything should be done *for* him. It really doesn't work that way. Mental health is something we do for ourselves, and no one else can do it for us.

So why don't we do it?

I suggest it is because we have forgotten how.

What does that mean?

Put simply, most people don't know *how* they are because they are not sure *who* they are, or what they are feeling.

Even the social chit-chat of every day undermines the idea. "How are you today?" "Fine! And you?" "Fine..." We've all seen people who claim to be 'fine' as their eyelids swell with unshed tears, their hands twist tortuously, and their entire demeanor signals pain and distress. The message that we send to each other, daily, is that everything is 'fine', and if it isn't, then we have to pretend that it is. Under such circumstances, we are not encouraged to look inwards. Ours is an outward-directed society, and we tend to judge each other by what we have rather than who we are. Even therapists tend to do it: "He has a big client base," "She has two books out." Rarely do we say that someone is happy as a first line of description.

Our estrangement from ourselves should not surprise us if we take a brief survey of our lives. When a child is born it is greeted with delight, usually, and its needs are attended to. Notice that the infant is not shy about expressing its needs. If the child is hungry, a piercing yell comes forth until the need is met. Likewise, damp diapers, heat, cold, and stomach ache - all produce a lusty complaint, and all are met with understanding and care. When the child begins to speak there is great excitement around those first words. All this is supportive and helpful as the child comes to terms with the world. Now skip ahead a few years to say fifth grade. The experience there is far more likely to be akin to that I had at school:

"Sit down and shut up."

"Speak only when you are spoken to."

And at my grandparents' home the dictum was the old Victorian idea: "children should be seen and not heard."

I am not being deliberately insensitive to the education system here when I suggest that most students expect to have teachers talk *at* them for large portions of the time. What could be a better example than the undergraduate at a major university who walks into a class of five hundred other students in a lecture hall? Or the visiting professor whose prepared speech is seen on closed circuit television?

Again and again the message is: sit down and shut up.

I would contend that for many people thinking is something that takes place during discussion, as they talk. Sometimes it is only as one begins to express one's ideas that one knows exactly what they are. How many times have we found ourselves in a discussion saying words to the effect that, "What I really meant to say is..."? Discussion can bring clarity, an exchange of ideas, a change of viewpoint. It doesn't occur if we sit down and shut up.

And that is, incidentally, exactly what I've been doing to you, here in this book. I've been filling the page with words, forcing you to be passive. See how easy it is to slip into that mode? Comfortable, too. When I have presented this information before groups in a class-room setting, it has always astonished me how easily those people slipped into being passive, listening, taking a few notes, being slightly bored. And yet the real materials of the class or seminar, the core of our reason for being there is they, themselves. We're all so used to not speaking our thoughts that we sometimes don't even know what they are any more.

What we have to do now is ask ourselves a few questions about who we are. Take a piece of paper, or write directly in this book. Take the time you need, and answer the questions in as many different ways as you can. For example, **who am I**? can be answered as:

I am a ...   male/female
I am a ...   student/teacher/accountant
I am ...   20/60/45 years old
I am ...   ambitious/timid/lonely.

And so on.
Do about ten of these.
When you have done that, try answering the question in its negative form.

I am not...

Write about a dozen of these.
Now take a look at your answers. Do you need to add anything? Go ahead. Add it. When you are finished look at the order in which you wrote your comments. Could you put beside each one a number, starting with 1, showing which is the most important to you? Take a look at the whole list. What does it tell you about you? Did you put your job as a higher priority than your personal connections? An example would be:

I am a Company Director   (1)
I am a mother   (2)

If, as in this example, your job rates more highly than your family commitments, what does that say about the balance in your life? Are there any tensions attached to this? I would imagine there would be plenty. The order in which your preferences occur is neither better nor worse than anyone else's, but it is yours, and deserves to be looked at.

Did you find as you went down the list that you became more personal or less so? Many people find they mention the less acknowledged part of themselves later, so "aspiring poet" may appear way down the list, although this is something the individual may value more highly than an activity that takes more time such as "P.T.A. Board Member". What are the items on your list that fit this category? What did you *forget* to mention? Why?

One man I worked with forgot to mention he was married since, he said, it was "just a fact of life, like my height or weight". It was a fascinating commentary upon his personal life, and later on as we worked together more fully, he began to see that his oversight pointed to an area of growing potential conflict, since his wife felt entirely abandoned by him. Another person, a woman, mentioned in her list, "I am beautiful, inside." Since she was extremely obese, the comment was both hopeful (she valued her spiritual qualities) and evasive of the fact that she was a compulsive eater, which she preferred to overlook.

In the list that begins, 'I am not' we can expect to see some comments about the more precise nature of the psyche. Sometimes people are not very kind to themselves here. "I am not easy to live with," wrote one woman, "I am not as mean as people think I am," wrote another. In each case the comment cries out to be examined further. If you *feel* you are not easy to live with, then it probably needs to be talked about, written about, looked at. And this is where you have to work. Write about it. It can be in a journal or on an old envelope, but keep it safe, for later reference. Talk about it to others, certainly. But write about it, you must.

Now taking a few steps back, what have we been doing? First of all, I placed you, the reader, in a submissive position by bombarding you with facts. I did this deliberately, because that is what a reader *expects*, for the most part, and it is certainly what groups that assemble together for self-exploration need, at least at first. In the group setting, as I give my opening statements, the participants in the group have their first chance to look at each other, size each other up, and size me up, as well. How threatening is this going to be, they ask themselves? The more I talk, the more they relax, confident that the center of emphasis is not themselves. For a moment they can all forget that what brought them to the room was the need to look inward, at themselves, that most daunting of all tasks.

When I draw attention to my ruse, it is not to negate the value of the information that has gone before. Quite to the contrary. My intention is merely to remind the participants of the real reason that brought us all there. The effect of this approach can be very satisfactory, for the individuals each know in their unconscious *exactly* why they are all there, and when reminded, tend to focus very sharply indeed on the activity at hand. You also, as reader, know why you picked up this book. You know you have work you need to do on yourself, but it is *work* after all, and it's always pleasurable to pretend it's not urgent, isn't it? I for one am no stranger to the delights of procrastination.

Once the mind is focused it is always a good idea to ask the most basic of questions, since they are often the most important. The question **who am I?** and the response, **I am**... tends to lead the participant into a discovery of the social roles he or she fulfills, often unwillingly. Every answer can convey a drama. For instance, one woman wrote: "I am nursemaid to my sick mother (unpaid)". Behind the statement one can immediately sense the feeling of being undervalued, "(unpaid)", as well as the issues of time, work and money that were involved, all of which seemed to indicate that a sense of dutiful love was crushing her. Talking about it with the group she wept at her dilemma, expressing her pain openly for the first time.

The reader working alone may not be able to experience that group sharing in the same way, which is why the writing of the emerging feelings can be so valuable. Since it is literally a sharing of one's self with one's self, it is an opportunity to meet oneself.

In the group setting, I have always found this exercise a remarkable way for group members to introduce themselves. The usual formal statements that I encourage group members to make round the room when we start tend to go like this:

"Hi, I'm Bill and I want to learn about myself."

After the exercise, however, all group members have a much more powerful sense of who Bill is, even if they forgot what his name was immediately after he originally spoke. In this way a group is able to make the acquaintance of its individual members, and also identify, without delay, some of the major issues that the individuals may be facing. This is vital, since I have participated in some groups that have spent several weeks failing to admit that there were any compelling reasons for gathering, and that has merely led to raised tensions and diminished expectations. Finally, the exercise lets group members know which others in the group have similar problems and concerns. This is important since those people will be the future gold-mines of information and insight for all. The person who really knows what child abuse is will be the person who was its victim. That person will be able to share wisdom with other victims, and in turn, reassure them that they are not alone. Knowing one is not alone is, in itself, empowering, quite apart from the added bonus of being able to share perceptions, and compare doubts and fears.

At the most basic level, such an exercise publicly acknowledges and reminds the individuals of the work to be done, and that it is ready to be tackled.

The reader, at this stage, may feel at a disadvantage with no group to fall back on. Don't despair. You may want to select someone with whom you can work together. It can even be done by writing to each other, so miles of distance are no problem. I have even come across students of mine who have worked in this way on e-mail. In many ways that can be a highly satisfactory way of working, although I believe each person should keep a copy of what he or she writes, for future reference. After all, our memories are fickle, and writing down what we think, or committing our ideas to tape, can be a valuable record. If you are reading this and feel the references to groups to be irksome, please consider for a moment why I have put them there. They are a form of feedback, telling you what you may expect, and letting you know that this is no sham. We are dealing with real pain and distress here.

Remember, sharing with a group may be exhilarating, terrifying, and cathartic, but the same effect can be achieved by the individual reader, you, writing about these things. As I wrote at the start, it is not vitally important that others understand you. Human beings are so complex that complete understanding is never really possible. What is important is that you begin to understand yourself. Until you do, you are like a person wandering around with a blindfold. Since you do not know which direction you need to go in, no one direction is any more important than any other.

The next topic that I'd like to deal with is **Naming**. Naming can be very important, since often our most frightening experiences are those which we cannot name. Hollywood has cashed in on this for decades. *They Came*

From Outer Space, by its very indefiniteness, thrilled audiences in the 1950s. Who or what is 'they' and what is 'outer space' anyway? Other horror movie titles include *The Thing*, *Alien 1,2*, and *3*, *It*, and even Samuel Beckett used the same idea for *The Unnameable*.

I'll give another example. If I'm driving along and my car starts to make unpleasant noises from under the hood, I worry. If I don't know what it is, I worry more. When I go to a mechanic and he says: "It's the hydraulic valve lifters," I know immediately that he knows what it is, and that it can be remedied if only I give him enough money. If, however, he shakes his head and tells me he has no idea what it is, he's never heard a sound like that before, and that it sounds serious, then my anxiety soars. I may lose sleep, even. In each case the final cost may be exactly the same, but in the second instance the uncertainty gives my fears a chance to make my life even more difficult.

Or let's take a more personal example. I feel ill and I go to the doctor. If he tells me I have 'flu and I should go to bed and take fluids, then I do as he says. I don't *feel* any better, and I don't have any medication, but after all, it's only 'flu and I'll have to get through it. If he looks at me and says he can't find anything wrong with me, then I'm likely to worry. My symptoms have not changed, but my mind imagines all sorts of dire things, and before I know it, I'm worried about cancer or worse. The fact that there is no label for me to feel secure with is what keeps me, and anyone else for that matter, anxious. To return to Hollywood, there's no logical reason why *They Came From Outer Space* should not be a hilarious comedy, involving delightful, intelligent extra-terrestrials who only want to make the world a better place to live in. If you ever see the movie, of course, you'll see that this is not quite the case.

Naming, then, helps us control information and feel secure with it. We quantify quality in the process. This is an essential aspect of therapy, since therapists often work with things that are not easy to categorize at first. Nightmares and dreams have many contradictory aspects, and only after a considerable number of dreams have been shared by client and therapist can one hope to come to any deep understanding of their meaning or significance. Yet nightmares can wake us, screaming, though we barely recall them, and dreams can haunt us for years as we try to puzzle them out. Part of the therapeutic process, in my view, has to be the naming of the event that gives rise to the fears and behaviors that are often the acting out of what the individual is afraid to acknowledge. An example may help here. I worked with one young man who had very wealthy parents who were also somewhat distant. Every Christmas and birthday they would give him a very expensive present. These he would immediately break, lose or smash, often 'accidentally'. When he 'accidentally' smashed the motorcycle they had given him one year, he was lucky to escape with only minor injuries. The next action was that he would then go and steal exactly the same item that had been destroyed. When we met he had an impressive juvenile criminal record, because he always seemed to get caught whenever he stole something. What he was acting out, in this way, was the fact that he wanted the things he was given, but he did not want his parents to give him these things. What he wanted from them was human love, attention, and recognition, not lavish gifts. The only way he could get attention, however, was by getting into trouble. That merely gave him negative attention, but what the heck, it was better than nothing, right? It was only when he was able to articulate the feeling that he both loved and resented his parents, that he needed and hated them, that he was able to stop the behavior. It was a long struggle to bring him to that 'naming' process.

Here, then, is a naming exercise you can do now. First, write your name.

Now, write your name as you would on a check.

Follow that with the signature you would use on a job application.

Below that sign your name as it would appear on a letter to your parents, or your older relatives.

Now, write your name as you would write it on a note to a loved one, or a friend your own age, or your best friend from college, say.

Now write it as you would to the significant other person in your life.

Now write out your full name any way you wish.

Take the last name and make it into a picture

Take as much time as you want. In group work, people have often spent twenty minutes or more on a drawing of this sort and the results have always been full of meanings, rich in detail.

What this exercise shows is the many different facets of our personality. Look at those signatures. Each one is you, but each is a different aspect of yourself, in a different context. The more exuberant you are, the more variation there is likely to be between the formal signature for a job interview, and the informal squiggle that many use as short-hand to loved ones. Those people who have minimal variation in the signatures may wish to ask why this is? Is it a desire to conform? A desire to avoid attention? The signature to one's parents or relatives can say a certain amount about the relationship involved, and that would be a fruitful area on which to base further discussions. Some people have nicknames that only exist in the family, and that make them feel slightly embarrassed when openly acknowledged. Those who do not have a healthy relationship with parents or relatives may tend to put that restraint, or constraint, into the signature, the size of the writing, and so on. Smaller, generally, indicates a more shy and retiring nature.

The same applies to the signature-picture. Large and energetic indicates an expansive nature. Small and confined indicates a lack of confidence. But more than this is *what* is drawn. This can be an important basis for further discussion. A young woman whose family had recently relocated drew a house around her signature, symbolizing for her the importance of a stable home to her identity. Naturally the permutations are almost endless. Look at your own signature-picture. It is you, as much as looking in a mirror is you. True, you probably didn't choose your name (few of us do), but each time you write it, you convey a vital aspect of yourself. Why do I say that? Consider, for a moment, how different our signatures all are. When we sign a check or a contract our signature is what authenticates the statement. It's as personal as our fingerprints. If they weren't different, we can be sure that the banks would long ago have thought of a better way of keeping our money safe. Forgers go to a vast amount of trouble to attempt to duplicate signatures, and the work is not easy. Certainly if you have ever attempted to copy someone else's signature you'll appreciate that.   These aspects of ourselves are distinctly ours. Graphologists and other handwriting experts are highly paid. Some will read your character and your future from your handwriting. Since this book is not concerned with graphology, I don't intend to spend much time on it except to say that it takes as axiomatic the fact that one's handwriting reflects one's selfhood. Do you remember in grade school practicing suitable signatures? I did, and Chris Baldwell who sat next to me spent hours perfecting his sense of his self-image in the squiggles he called his signature. In each, he was, effectively, drawing an abstract picture of himself.

Here are some examples for your to consider. I have used my own signature since, obviously, people I have worked with do not want to be discussed by name in this book as that would violate confidentiality.

What can one say about my signatures, here? The first thing is that they are all a good size, positioned firmly on the center of the page, if a little too far up. That's me all over - I leave a little too much time or space for many events (in this case the 'event' is the picture) that I'm looking forward to. Conversely, I never allow enough time and space for things I don't like to do.   I'm the original person who hopes to do 14 errands in 15 minutes, but if I have a dinner party, I'll plan days ahead. The snake, bounding along, mirrors my eagerness to get on with these exercises and get to know people. It indicates both my excitement (since I usually do the exercise at the start of a group's series of sessions) and my future need, in group work, to be super-sensitive to all around me. As the Bible tells us, the serpent was "the subtlest creature of all the field" -- and that's what I feel I have to be, some-times, in order to understand individuals.

I stress this example because any response to any exercise will have at least two values. The first is what is being felt *now*, and the second is what the deeper concerns are one might have about who one *is*. In group work I am a little sneaky, since I've done the exercises before, so I feel a bit like a snake, I suppose, because I have that unfair advantage. That is the deep value. The surface value is merely eager anticipation, as seen in the bounding forward movement. At another level, I have to say that person-ally, I feel the movement of the snake has a great deal to do with my sense that this is an exciting time in my life and that I am moving rapidly forward in many ways.

So here is a brief synopsis of the analysis of these drawings. The draw-ing will exist on three levels. The first level is 'here and now'. The draw-ing's actual look will depend on how the drawer is feeling right as he or she draws. If he or she has a headache, indigestion, or is bored, the drawing will mirror that, certainly. This could lead to important questions, also. If the person has a headache, is it because of a bad day? What caused the day to be stressful? ... And so on.

The second level is the *content* of the drawing, rather than the execution of it. What does the drawing *show*? One man produced sketches of a figure with a sword stabbing horses. Clearly the violent, possibly sexual, nature of the drawing begged for further questions about what seemed to be the man's simmering anger. Others have drawn sketches of hills with walkers or ski-ers, showing scenes of pleasure and relaxation, in which the content indi-cated memories of happy times and a longing for them to return once again.

The third level is the *action* of the picture. Is this a static scene or a dy-namic scene? This would tend to indicate whether the individual sees her/himself as moving forward, as developing, or as settled, fixed and un-moving. There is no hard and fast rule here - or anywhere, really - as to what this may mean for an individual, since stasis is often necessary and reassuring. However, it is worth noting that those who tend to use static images of themselves in such drawings are more likely to be stuck in a rut, or looking for security. When working with the severely depressed, static images abounded. The implication seems to be that people suffering from depression are less likely to see themselves as capable of change, and therefore, as static.

If this all sounds rather vague, do not despair. Until you have done several exercises you will not be able to look at yourself as an outsider might and attempt to unravel the meaning of the images. It is in the cumulative effect of such work that the value lies. One picture of a badly drawn snake is not enough to give anyone much insight into who I am, for example, but it may yield sufficient clues to make some educated guesses later, when connected to other exercises.

Standing back from the exercises, you may wish to speculate about what they tell you about yourself, taking time to write down the ideas that come to you, asking questions. Remember, this section has been about the activity of **naming**, and you have been looking at your own name, considering who you are.

Naming is not always straightforward in our cultures. At confirmation, Christian children (and adults) often take a name that is supposed to be a saint's name, indicating in that way which saint's life the confirmed intends to emulate. Baptism is in itself a symbolic taking of a new, washed-clean life, and of a new name. Since many churches practice infant baptism, the chance to change or choose a new name for oneself is diminished. In the United States it is legally possible to change one's name, should one wish to do so, but in many places one's name is simply given one. Whether it comes to be a burden later, or not, is rarely considered.

Think for the moment of the person with an unusual name or a name that carries some sort of stigma. Consider the case of the Marine Sergeant, an American, born with the surname Hitler. He resolutely refused to change it, though he served in the Second World War. At a different level, how about the man who grows up called, say John Smith IV? The familial expectation that he will fill his father's shoes would seem to be written into his name. What pressure does that put on him to conform?

Consider your own name, now, and write it down. Then complete the following phrases, in writing.

My name is _____

I like my name because _____
_____
_____

I don't like my name because _____
_____
_____

If I chose a name it would be _____

Now I think _____
_____
_____
_____

Now I feel _____
_____
_____
_____

The name discussion is an important one because it can shed light on one's own sense of being, of identity, and contrast it to what one's family seems to want one to be. Choosing one's own name can also be revealing. Some tribes of plains Indians have a custom of giving a tribe member three names. One is the family name, a surname; one is the birth name - a sort of Christian name; and the third name is not chosen until puberty, a little like a confirmation name. The idea is that this third name should describe the specific attributes and talents of the individual. That name should be based in the person's strengths so that in a time of crisis he or she can recall that name in order to recall exactly where the character is strongest and use that energy. An example would be, perhaps "He-who-runs-fast". That would describe the person's quality and his way of doing things. In a crisis such a person would be reminded that his talent lies in moving swiftly rather than, say, in going through a slow negotiation process. The idea would be that if a person acts according to his or her talents and strengths, then that person will be authentic and act effectively. It is when we try to be who we are not that we wind up in trouble.

Looking at your replies in this last exercise, do you feel your name really reflects who you *are*? In my experience people rarely feel their given names to be perfectly apt. Many feel proud to have their names, the names of admired and loved relatives, and hope to live up to those names. Some people are named after Biblical characters and take great pride in that. How do you feel about your name?

It's not an idle question. One woman I worked with discovered in her thirties that she had been named after one of her father's mistresses with whom he had been having a passionate affair when his wife became pregnant. Obviously such circumstances produced mixed feelings about her name and sense of self worth, as well as emotions about her parents. And this brings us to the entire discussion of women's names which have, traditionally, been lost when the woman married. More and more women keep their names these days after marriage, but what about the surnames of any children they might have? The relaxing of traditions brings choices that may be difficult, especially if the woman marries, produces children who take the father's surname, and then divorces with some bitterness. That is just one example, but a not uncommon one.

The real tension of the exercise, however, will tend to collect around the last two items; **Now I think**... **Now I feel**.

In group work this has often proved to be very emotionally charged. After working through several exercises like this, asking someone how he or she *feels*, and getting that person to write it down, can make it seem to many that they have no option but to tell the truth about their feelings. Yet the question is open. One could choose to reply: "now I feel hungry" or "cold", after all. The question asks us to make a choice between the purely factual and the emotionally important. Which did you choose? Often the purely factual statement indicates that the person is avoiding facing the issues, or that the person simply doesn't understand what's going on. Careful questions may be needed here. After all, not knowing can be a major psychological defense to a perceived threat. The cliché that springs to mind is of the fifth grader in the principal's office being asked why he or she did something. "I don't know," comes the reply over and over. And sometimes the child does not know in the sense that he or she is unable to give a short, concise answer such as the Principal is looking for. It is not an easy question to reply to: what do you feel, now?

   With this we return to the discussion with which we started the chapter, that it is difficult to know who we are and what we are feeling, and that unless we know these things we can find ourselves confused, adrift and in despair. This has never been more important than it is today. In my grandfather's time, in Switzerland where he grew up, he knew very firmly what his family ties were, and what the townspeople of his tiny country town expected people to do. He had the choice to conform or leave. He conformed, aware that he was directly related to almost half the town, and had been through school with everyone his own age. At every turn, he knew who he was and was reminded as to who he was expected to be. Sixty years later, I, his grandson, live in a town with no blood relatives, my parents and other relatives are all several hours plane-ride away, and the people I know here I have only been acquainted with for a few years, at most. Many of them have different religious beliefs and cultural expectations. My point is that without the outward reassurances that my grandfather had, my generation, and future generations, have to be far more assured about who we are *internally*. The media, through the all-pervasive television, tell us that the ideal of female attractiveness should be about 20 years old, wear a certain style of clothes, and so on. Yet, I know that this type of woman is not my ideal. For one thing she is only half my age. The television and the media do tell us who we should be as far as they are concerned - which is in order to sell us certain products, many of which we may not need. We are continuously bombarded by messages telling us not who we *are* (like my grandfather's townspeople) but how we are not managing to measure up to the ideal unless we purchase a certain product, move to a certain place, act a certain way ... and so on. And next season the message changes. We have, therefore, to be careful to find out who we are, or we risk becoming nothing at all.
   The image that I see most often is the one I call the geek in the muscle-car. The young man has been convinced that he has to have a big, expensive, fast car, probably at vast price with a repayment plan he can barely manage, and is surprised to find he is no more attractive or successful than before. He has the outer trappings, but not the inner substance. Now, this is not to say that the geek can never have substance. He can, and does. But he has to look within to find it, and its price may not be monetary in the same way the car payments are. There is a price to be paid. It includes honesty, determination and an investment of time.

That's what you and I, reader, are doing with this book. We're looking inside to see who *exactly* is inside.

In this section I've emphasized the ideas of naming, of identifying thoughts and feelings, and writing them down. Why is it important for us to write them down? Here is an answer that may help to explain this.

In conventional therapist-client relations, one of the largest issues that initially faces the client is that of trust. The fear is that if the client really says what is on his or her mind then the therapist may be appalled or hostile. This issue can take many months to resolve, during which time the client is usually in some pain. One young man I worked with took many months before he could admit that he hated his abusive father - and was then horrified at what he had said. I would suggest that he and others like him could have saved a great deal of pain and anxiety if the initial realization of that hatred could have been expressed privately, safely, on paper. As it was, he spent months acting out his distress by aggressive acts towards older male figures in his life who were *not* his father. This, for him, was the only way to express what he was feeling because, despite being highly articulate, he could not bring himself to talk about his problem. Once he did so, the behavior changed rapidly. Unfortunately by that time he had a string of criminal charges against him. My contention would be that had this man had a safe way of addressing his anxieties he could have at least shortened the time span in which he was vulnerable to his delinquent behavior.

Writing, after all, can help us in obvious ways. Consider the pocket diary. I'm lost without mine. It reminds me where I should be and when, and in so doing, it removes from me a huge amount of anxiety about what I'm supposed to be doing. To say that it keeps me sane is a cliché, but in a real sense, it does so. Shopping lists work the same way. Without them I return home and discover to my intense annoyance that I've forgotten several vital items. The shopping list saves me time and exasperation, and helps to keep me calm. At night, if I have a busy day the next day, I have two options, one is to take a sleeping tablet and hope that my racing mind will slow down, the other, which works far better, is to write a "to do" list just before I roll over and sleep. It clears my mind. Another example of the beneficial effects of writing might be the letter full of raging emotions that is never sent. One can write through the anger and arrive at a calmer place. Many of these feelings might be embarrassing if spoken out loud, or even harmful. It is a poor idea, usually, to tell one's boss exactly what one thinks of him or her, but then, what does one do with those feelings? A safe place to put them would be on paper. One may feel like throttling colleagues, but it is unwise to attempt to do so; the fantasy needs to be acknowledged and then left behind. These are all examples of the usefulness of writing in keeping us sane.

I am not suggesting that writing can supplant therapy entirely. That would be naive. What I am suggesting is that writing can be used as a powerful therapeutic tool to be applied either on its own as a mental health maintenance technique, or alongside therapeutic counseling as a way of coming to terms more efficiently with distress. One of the remarkable things about people is their ability to forget and avoid. The raging toothache disappears when the nervous patient arrives at the dentist's chair. People say things and then deny having said them, often actually believing their own denial. A client can leave a therapist's office and ten minutes later have 'forgotten' everything that was said. We forget who we were and what we did, all too rapidly. That is one reason why I enjoy photograph albums so much. I look at them and say, "Did I ever dress like that?" "Why did I have such a strange haircut?" And I marvel at the things that we all accepted as usual only a few years earlier. Photographs can remind us of what we choose to gloss over. Just similarly do diaries function. Good gracious, we say to ourselves reading a journal of some previous time, did I ever feel like that? Well, yes. We did. And often it is a very good idea to be reminded about those feelings. We cannot pretend, reading those old entries, that we never really cared for those people. By writing it down, we have proof that the feeling existed, and therefore, we can respect our feelings, and gain a deeper knowledge of who we were, and are.

A friend of mine recently came across some old 16mm movies made of him when he was 11. Curious, he set up a projector and watched them. It was, he admitted, a sobering experience. To begin with, he was able to see, first hand, what a conceited child he had been, and how he had treated his siblings. Second, he was able to see some aspects of the way his entire family responded to each other. He spent a long time thinking about this and came gradually to a better understanding of how his own family had been (rather than how he thought they had been), and how that had affected all their lives. It also made him look anew at his own children, and reassess how he acted with them. It was, he says, very moving. With the arrival of the video camera as a household item I suspect that in the future we will see many such home movies being used in therapy as a way of reappraising the past.

Children in foster homes in several London boroughs are, today, often given the chance to construct a "Book of Life", in which the child visits the major places that have made a contribution to his to her life. In this way the child care worker will take a photograph of, say, the child standing outside the hospital of birth, and at the door of the first home, the first school, and so on. The pictures are then placed in an album for the child. The effect is to reclaim time that has been forgotten and straighten out confused memories. Social workers report that the books help to give the child or young adult a stronger sense of belonging, of identity.

I mention both of these examples because the 'writing' can be achieved in many ways, not all of them involving paper and pencils. Many people report having good success with tape recorders and video cameras for the recording of events and ideas. Personally, I believe that the most profound work of self-exploration can only be done with the help of an audience response - a friend, a counselor - and that one's most critical audience is likely to be oneself. One can best stand outside oneself, in my view, by reviewing one's own writing. There it is, what one has written. One cannot disregard it. In a world where it is difficult to be listened to, or acknowledged, one can at least acknowledge oneself.

This is why I call this activity therapeutic writing.

CHAPTER TWO

In the preceding chapter we worked on names as a way of considering who we are, and we tried to make sense of things that are often taken for granted, such as signatures. Each signature was like a miniature self portrait of how we want that aspect of ourselves to be seen by the world. It's a very studied, deliberate portrait. What I'd like to do now is move to something looser.

When working with a group I always like to allow the first section of time for feedback from the previous session. It serves to remind the group about what we did, why we did it, and what it might have meant for them. Usually the group is extremely attentive in the first set of exercises, and it is always a good idea to remind everyone how seriously they took themselves at the time. People really work hard in some of these sessions, but because it is work done on one's own psyche it often may not feel like conventional work. This leads some participants to think the process is easy and simple. Others become bemused when something so unlike their usual activities is praised as 'work'. That is part of the reason I insist on reflection papers being written after each session, so that what was experienced can be recorded. To give an example - the first time I made a parachute descent from an airplane I giggled all the way down to the -thump- ground. I knew immediately I had landed that I had to go again, because I had been unable to grasp the experience fully the first time. So I got back to the airstrip, packed up the 'chute and went back for a second drop. This time, the second time, I was able to feel all the apprehension, all the sense of fragility, and to marvel at my own foolhardiness - or was it courage? The second time was certainly not the same experience, since that time I knew I was

scared, but it enabled me to know, to feel all the emotions that had been hidden behind my giggles.   Yes, I was frightened, but also the experience became immeasurably more wonderful for me as I heard the wind whistling in
the cords and felt, rather than heard the calm after the blasting noise of the
aero-engines. It remains with me as one of the magical moments of my life.
I never did a third jump.

The paper - the chance to write about the previous work in the group -
that is a version of the second jump. If you are working alone with this
book, that is to say not with another person or a group, the paper will be
essential, and each re-reading of it a chance to reassess.

I'd like now to do something different, something with some silliness.
Here is a poem you may recognize: *Jabberwocky* by Lewis Carroll. Kenneth Koch is the inspiration for this exercise.

Read the poem; it's about a monster.

'Twas brillig and the slithy toves
Did gyre and gimble in the wabe
All mimsy were the borogroves
And mome raths outgrabe

"Beware the Jabberwock, my son,
The jaws the bite the claws the catch,
Beware the Jub-Jub bird and shun
The frumious Bandersnatch."

He took his vorpal blade in hand,
Long time the manxome foe he sought,
So rested he by the Tumtum tree
And stood a while in thought.

And as in uffish thought he stood
The Jabberwock with eyes of flame
Came whiffling through the tulgey wood
And burbled as it came!

One-Two, One-Two and through and through
His vorpal blade went snicker-snack!

He left it dead and with it's head
He went galumphing back.

"And hast thou slain the Jabberwock?
Come to my arms my beamish boy!
Oh frabjous day, Callooh, Callay!"
He chortled in his joy.

'Twas brillig and the slithy toves
Did gyre and gimble in the wabe,
All mimsy were the borogroves
and mome raths outgrabe.

Try out those weird words. 'Slithy' - what does that convey to you? 'Wimble' and 'wabe' have a suggestiveness also. Read them out loud and hear the words. Now, close your eyes for a moment. Think of the words. Take out some clean paper. Draw the Jabberwock.

Take all the time you need: try not to talk to anyone as you draw. Don't look at anyone else's before you've finished.

When doing this exercise in groups, I have seldom had anyone need less than 20 minutes to do the drawing. This I understand as the degree of intensity with which participants attack this assignment.

When all the drawings are complete, I ask the participants to place their Jabberwock in front of them and say a few words about it. This is often accompanied by questions such as: "How big is it?" "Is it male or female?" and, "What are those things?" The last question is often necessary since many people are not good at drawing and certain objects need to be explained. Sometimes the discussions begin immediately, but on the whole, most people are on their first parachute jump, here, and are not sure what they have produced.

If you are working alone, take the time to write down what the picture shows, and explain the action. What is the jabberwock doing? What is happening?

In group work, when all the pictures have been seen, and remain on view for all, then comes the time for some interpretative comments. The comments I will make here can be applied to your picture if you are working

alone. Write down your responses to them, and what thoughts they produce.

I will start by making a few general observations. The pictures that have
been produced will depend on many things. The first thing is the cultural
background of the artist. Some people draw versions of things that they
have seen in movies. (The Wookie from *Star Wars*, or the Monty Python
version of *Jabberwocky*) and this will cloud the particular vision of the artist. Knowing that, however, we can reach behind the culturally determined
layer and begin to see some useful information. One man drew a Bugs
Bunny-type figure and defended his choice by saying, "I never learned to
draw anything else!" In his case the defensiveness he brought to the exercise
threatened to erase its meaning for him. Luckily, by seeing the creatures the
others drew, he was able to understand what was going on. Although the
exercise was not a great success for him, he could see that it worked for
others. He then went home and re-drew his Jabberwock - neatly dismantling
his claim that he could not draw anything else.

Given that we have to work carefully, it is as well to realize that these
drawings are often very personal. It is frequently very threatening for people to have their drawings scrutinized, but I want to emphasize at this point
that this is not merely a silly parlor game for damp afternoons. We are
touching on important things here. Three days after one session a woman in
her mid-40s came to see me and begged to be allowed to leave the group.
The reason she gave was that she had been unable to sleep since producing
her drawing, and she was very frightened. She had already scheduled sessions with a former therapist, she said, but she could not keep coming to my
sessions. Naturally I was concerned, but hardly surprised. These drawings
can be very powerful, since they can, if used correctly, tap into the deepest
parts of our psyches. These monsters we draw could be seen as a version,
an approximation, of our own personal monsters, of our deep fears, or of
our anger.

What does this mean? Since the poem is a nonsense poem that uses invented words, we can give whatever meaning we want to the words; and we
do. One woman who drew the Jabberwock in the instant of having its head
severed had, it turned out, been that very day to her court hearing for divorce. The anger, the split, all were in the picture, not surprisingly. That
picture referred primarily to her experience *now*, rather than to, say, a
childhood trauma. She was certain the monster she had drawn was her ex-
husband. Another woman, divorced a year earlier, showed a dinosaur in a

desert looking lost, and an eel swimming away across a lake. "That," she said, "is my husband. I'm the eel, swimming to safety." The figures were tiny on the page, making the dinosaur look even more lost, alone and ready for extinction. Two young men who both had considerable anger towards their fathers, each drew large and impressive monsters, but their emphasis was on the small boy with the 'vorpal blade' who was ready to do battle.

Often, to avoid placing a group member in the spotlight, I will use my own drawing as an example. Here it is.

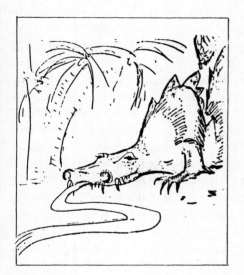 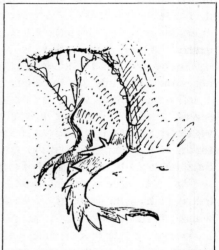

The first question to ask is: where is the drawing on the page? Mine, as you can see, started central to the page and then I needed a second page added on. This would tend to indicate that the problems the monster brings are larger and more complex than at first I realized. Since I am aware the monster is a symbol of the relationship with my father and with authority figures - I always think of the monster as male - the space issue is important. By comparison, one young woman drew me a picture of a creature with a huge head with a tiny body, surrounded by tiny houses. She knew immediately I talked about monsters who it was, interrupting me to say,

"That's my mother! That's the way she *is*. She never stops talking..." Her mother was quite simply the biggest issue in her life, the largest object in her mental landscape, and appeared as such on the page.

Another woman, with two small children and a disabled husband, drew a teddy bear type creature in one crowded corner of an otherwise empty page, surrounding this inoffensive monster with Jub jub birds, Tumtum trees, shrubs and so on. Gentle questioning led her to the point where she could say that the monster was, in fact, herself. Always giving way to others, she felt hemmed in, cornered by the demands of her family, and that their love was imprisoning her by being expressed only as demands on her. A young man drew an empty landscape of rocky desert, with only the vorpal blade in it. No Jabberwock at all. Afterwards he was able to say that this was pre-cisely his problem - he hid his feelings and anxieties. "I buried them in the desert," he said.

Young women, I find, tend to produce drawings that look like teddy bears and are totally non-threatening in appearance. This does not mean the exercise has failed. Often, I find that such drawings are pictures of them-selves, since they may see themselves as friendly, relatively harmless, and yet under threat (by the boy in the poem). Such pictures seem to indicate a feeling of puzzlement about the demanding and dangerous world we live in. Such images articulate a level of fear about their future.

This is usually the point at which a group member or two will say that this is making no sense at all, so let me use my own drawing to illustrate what is going on.

Whenever I do this exercise - and bear in mind one can repeat the exer-cises, knowing what they convey, and still learn new things - I produce the same sort of dragon. In previous years he (and I'm sure he is male) has been flying through the air, vicious, angry, about half a mile long. Recently, I've envisioned him half asleep in a cave, but he's still too big to fit on one page. Here is what I think this may say about me. The dragon is, as I have said, about authority figures in general and in particular about my feelings to-wards my father. He was in the Air Force for many years (hence the flying) and because I was away at boarding school he always felt distant. He is also, sometimes, quick tempered, a fact that he finds hard to suppress, and I have had some difficulty approaching him over the years. The picture is partly him, and partly all the male figures I've had difficulty dealing with as a result of my own unreconciled feelings about my father. I never really learned how to deal with the main authority figure in my life, because we were often in different countries altogether. We still are. I then asked myself how I would kill this Jabberwock, if I were the boy in the poem. And immediately, I knew. Such a monster cannot be attacked head-on. Instead I knew I would have to wait until that long neck was extended and attack from the side. It seems to me that this is exactly the way I tend to work in a conflict. I do not usually face it head-on, I will sidestep, outflank my adversary. I always have. In a sense this exercise is an example of side-stepping, since it encouraged me to see my monster in a new light and reassess the problem. I am attracted to these exercises, and to writing this book, because I am well-trained in taking the side-step. I've done it all my life. I simply never realized it fully until I did this exercise. So, ask yourself, how will you deal with your monster? Attack it? Ambush it? Care for it?

In this drawing I for the first time drew the Jabberwock dozing in a cave. What could this mean? Several things. My relationship with my father has calmed now to a more relaxed and loving one, and part of it has to do with his age (he's 77 at this time), part of it has to do with the fact that I've finally 'settled down' in his eyes. I have bought my first home, and he has visited, feeling quite relaxed. He no longer feels he has to prod me along to be someone in the world, since I've quietly insisted on being myself. His caring, which I sometimes experienced as his anger at me, now shines through. After all, it is difficult not to feel criticism as an angry comment even if it is intended to help. The dragon has accepted the home. The dragon is not just my father, neither is it my fears of him, instead it is the creature that came into being when I saw what I took to be anger, and added my own angry response to the mix. It is the potentially destructive aspect of our relationship.

This is what the dragon, the Jabberwock, can mean. It can depict the harmful part of a relationship between two people, if we are willing to look at it that way. I am certainly not saying my father is a monster. He isn't. What I'm saying is that some of his behavior to me seemed frightening and raised fear and antagonism in me many years back, so that I envisioned that part of our relationship in this way.

Now, look at your own drawing. Where is it on the page? How big is it? These are indicators of how strong and urgent you are letting the problem (and even a friendly monster is a problem, let's face it) be in your life. How dangerous is it? A woman who felt her mother constantly monitored her every move drew a creature with scores of eyes. A man who drew a friendly vast dinosaur that clumsily trod on things later expressed the fact that he felt his father simply had no idea who he was, and inadvertently de-valued all he did.

What sort of pen strokes were used? Are they faint and sketchy or hard and dark? Harder and darker tends to convey a sense of definiteness, and of anger. Use this information to establish the mood when you were drawing.

What other figures are present? Who are they? Are there more 'extra' figures than anything else? How *crowded* is this picture? Crowded pictures will tend to indicate a busy, overcrowded life in which the individual may not find space to be him or herself.

Often it is the less than expert draftsperson who produces the most re-vealing drawing. Those with artistic training may be hung up on technique, and so the beauty of the picture becomes an issue. Bear in mind that in this work it is not the quality of the art that is at issue, but rather the ability of the exercise to express what had been previously unexpressed. It is unlikely that anyone in the average group will produce a poem to equal Yeats or a picture to hang beside DaVinci's. We are less concerned with the product than with the process. My own picture is no thing of beauty, but it tells me a great deal about myself.

Again, look at your picture. In any group I can make suggestions about the issues these pictures may raise, but it really does not matter if I can in-terpret them. What matters is what you understand and learn from them. I refer to my own picture in groups because I do not wish to put anyone else into the spotlight against his or her will, but often my personal confessions will help others to think, to see, and to talk.

As I say, it's a powerful exercise, and, to paraphrase a colleague of mine, we're playing with real money on the table. For that reason, it is vital to allow enough time for closure on this exercise. When I do this with a group I always leave enough space for group members to voice their fears, ideas and insights. If you are working alone it is a good idea to allow a space of time to think and wind down after the drawing. Since the drawing is very likely to contain information about conflicts with parents and family, it is only sensible not to visit or phone those people immediately afterwards, when the feelings may be still a little raw.

This brings me to a note about timing. It is important to start at the same time, and end at the correct time when working with a group. When dealing with personal material some participants may become overly anx-ious if they feel the group is not going to end on time. One should, therefore, always allow enough time so that it is not necessary to hurry anyone along.

Monsters are in our psyches for many reasons. When we dream them, we usually imagine them as big rather than, say ant-like. King Kong is far more compelling than Killer Bees, it seems, and dinosaurs are perennial favorites with children. One might expect a five or six-year-old, about three feet tall, to be terrified of the life-sized models and fossils that adorn our museums, displays, and even some parks. Quite the opposite. The stegosaurus outside the Natural History Museum in Washington, D.C. is a big favorite, as are elephant rides at zoos. By comparison, lions and bears are hardly in the same league. I suspect that for children, who regularly become besotted with dinosaurs, it is a vast relief to realize that there really are such things as monsters, but that they are safely dead, now, thank you. Almost every child who has fears of the creature hiding under the bed at night, of the ghoul in the coat closet, of the vampires in the attic, and so on, has no fear at all of dinosaurs, 'terrible lizards' as their name literally means. Eight-year-olds I know can name and identify up to a dozen different dinosaurs, but can't tell a sycamore from an oak, or a Ford from a Buick. The monsters mean something to them, which is why they are captivated by them. Children know about fear, and about monsters. They also know that these monsters, at least, are safely under control.

Children have always been entertained by stories about monsters being vanquished. Whether it be the Big Bad Wolf or the Giant in *Jack and the Beanstalk* the correlation is exactly the same. To small children all adults are monster-like in size, and the ones that are most influential in their lives are their parent-figures. When Jack steals back his father's treasure and kills the Giant he is doing more than his father could in confronting the monster. He is, in a sense, outwitting both his father and the angry paternal authority embodied in the Giant. All this is a way of saying that we should not be surprised to see that many of the drawings of giants and monsters produced in this exercise will have to do with conflicts with parents. That is why it is important to identify the sex of the monster, since that will help to identify the parent figure who is most problematic.

A second exercise that can be done that follows up on the idea of parent-child conflicts is as follows. This may take some time and is best done at home alone. Groups can be set this as a 'homework' assignment.

Using magazines and paper, prepare a collage around the topic of the family dinner.

Now write about it.

One of the extraordinary things about family meals is that because the family is together in the same room all the tensions that exist between them tend to emerge and be expressed in terms of food. This is certainly why for some families Thanksgiving, Christmas and Sunday lunch seem to be times of great stress, and why some people dread those occasions. The collages can be used as information in themselves and as spring boards for further discussion and writing. One young woman related how she had come into the family dining room one evening and had discovered that her father had nailed a loaf of bread to the ceiling. There was nothing else to eat. The food was there, but it was neither very appetizing nor accessible. Her father, it would seem, had certain strong feelings about providing for his family. The 'breadwinner' had said, in effect, 'That's all I'm prepared to do, and you can scramble for it!' This sort of information about the family tensions is well worth further exploration in writing and indeed as the woman began to write she began to recall more and more evidence of the tensions that had haunted the family dinner table. This allowed her to see, for the first time, what her parents' relationship had been, and how it had affected her.

Another woman was unable to make a collage at all. She had cooked for herself and her alcoholic mother from a very early age, terrified that the social workers would put her into an orphanage if it were ever discovered that her mother was incapable of providing food for her, she said. Now she hated the thought of even producing a collage of meal times. A third woman related tales of her father's anger. If he was dissatisfied with something he simply tipped the table over, smashing all the plates, and ending the meal.

I mention these examples specifically because eating disorders are very common amongst women, and since they are essentially life-threatening, it is as well for us to confront the possibility of them as early as possible in our work. What are your recollections of meal times? Did you get enough to eat? Did you feel you were forced to eat too much? If you have ever starved yourself or found yourself eating and then vomiting on a regular basis, you may need help. Don't delay. This book can do a vast amount, but you will certainly need more direct guidance in greater detail if you have an eating disorder.

When you think back to those family meal times, what do you feel? What did you feel then? A good technique is to search out a photograph of yourself as a child. Place it somewhere you can see it easily. Pin it to a wall, or paste it in your diary. As you remember family occasions at the dinner table (and you will remember many, I'm certain) look at the photograph and ask yourself, "What did that child think of all this at the time? What was he/she feeling?" Not surprisingly this lets us look back on events that we may have discarded as merely strange, and it puts us in contact with the feelings of the child. The woman who told of her father tipping over the table laughed about it as she related the story, but when she looked at the photograph of herself she was able to identify her feelings of panic and terror that she had sought for so long to suppress. Identifying the feelings, naming them, allowed her gradually to move beyond the events, and to recognize that her father's behavior was neither usual nor healthy.

This brings us to another part of the same topic that has to do with naming, which I mentioned in chapter one. Many people don't know what they feel about these events as they describe them. It is not uncommon to find people telling horror stories like those above and when asked what they feel about those events, they simply reply, "Nothing", or "I don't know." A wise therapist I came across had a technique for this. She had a large board on which were written several dozen words, all of them concerning the emotions. The board had words like, sad, happy, angry, raging, depressed, weepy, glum, elated ... written all over it. Clients were encouraged to point to a word that they felt expressed their mood after they had told of an episode in their lives. She reported that at first many clients could barely do this, because they had shut down the emotions, they had stopped themselves from feeling. Gradually, as the sessions went forward, they would become more adept at identifying their emotions. Once again we are in the realm of Naming.

Make a board like that for yourself. Add words to it when you need to. When you think of a portion of your life, try to find a word that matches what you feel about that period now. Then take a look at the photograph of yourself as a child, and try to imagine what the child would have chosen to say. Write about it.

CHAPTER THREE

Now that we have drawn and, possibly, identified the Jabberwock in our lives there can be little doubt that we are dealing with potentially vital material. Remember - and I'll keep stressing this point - that it is not always necessary for another person to explain your actions to you, or even understand you at all. The eminent therapist Carl Rogers pioneered the approach to the client in which, on the whole, he refrained from making any comment on what was said during the counseling sessions. He would encourage the client to speak, but would not intervene other than by using certain techniques to encourage the client to say more. One of these was merely to repeat the last phrase the client had uttered before falling silent. Whatever the disadvantages of this approach (it does not work very well with clients who will not speak at all, for example, but then such clients need different stratagems) the advantage seems to be that the client is the one who is made to face him or her self, and thus to understand the particular issues that are in question.

It's up to you.

One always has choices, after all. In one group, I had a young man who was very macho, and very highly defended. He was a humorist and always undercut anything he said by turning it into a joke. This certainly lightened the tone of the group, but it actually prevented him from facing his self-destructive anger. At a certain point he found it safer to respond to the exercises by being dishonest, inventing episodes, and lying. What was remarkable was the patience extended to him by the rest of the group. All of them could sense that he was being less than honest, but all seemed to realize that to challenge him about it would force him to hold on to his evasion even more tightly. The exercises were not successes for him, yet, in a strange way, they were not failures, either. He began to realize he simply was not ready for the work required of him. No one but oneself can ever say when one is ready. As you read this, you may feel apprehensive yourself. That is not a bad sign. But if you find after several chapters that this is not working for you, don't despair. Put the book down. Return to it a year from now. You and this book may simply not be ready for each other yet.

On the other hand, you may feel these exercises to be silly, too simple, too naive to consider. I would urge you to think again. Often the most important questions are those that seem the simplest. Whether we look at the devastatingly simple question to Saul in the Bible: "Quo Vadis?" "Where are you going?" or the complexity of the question "Who are you?", it can hardly be claimed that the simple question is always facile.

Here is an exercise that I call 'complete the sentence', since it starts with a series of statements that are to be completed. Here they are. Complete them one at a time. In group work I usually read them aloud and get everyone to write down the response before moving on to the next item. This prevents people from preparing 'suitable' answers for the statements further down the list. It is important to proceed through these in the correct order, and at a gentle pace, gradually slowing towards the end to allow more writing time. The first statement probably needs no more than 15 seconds before moving to the next.

As big as a _____

As square as a_____

As round as_____

As flat as_____

As yellow_____

As tall _____

-Pause-

This room is a_____

This town is_____

This activity is_____

This is _____

Now, I think _____

_____

_____

Now, I feel _____

_____

_____

Look at what you wrote. Clearly the exercise is geared towards the last line. What do you feel? How easy or difficult was it to deal with that question? What did you write? The exercise is arranged to give each person choices. One can choose to answer each incomplete sentence in a very neutral way. It is possible to write: "Now, I feel hungry/thirsty/cold..." Yet, very few people ever opt to stay at that literal level, and many become very imaginative, very quickly.

The exercise is based on similes (something is *like* something else) and metaphors (something *is* something else). The first part is designed to be non-threatening. If, for example, I say that my friend is behaving *like* a pig it implies that he isn't usually that badly behaved. If I say he *is* a pig it suggests that his character has undergone a more radical change. Just similarly the questions move from simile to metaphor, and thus probe deeper.

The first items, 'As big as a ...', 'As square as a ...', 'As round as...', 'As flat as...' all invite cliché, and usually get it. These are safe questions and produce predictable results for the most part. But notice that 'As round as' and 'As flat as' drop the indefinite article, leaving room for abstract answers to enter. One man who wrote "As big as a house"; "As square as a square"; "As round as a ball", suddenly produced "As flat as my relationship with my wife." Suddenly we were directly in contact with an imaginative leap that had brought us face to face with one of his major issues. Usually though, it's not until we reach 'As yellow...' and 'As tall...' that things really open up. My two most memorable contributions were "As yellow stalks of corn wave desperate hands at the sun" and "As Tall as God". Certainly in each case we had reached powerful individual emotions that needed to be talked about.

After the pause come the metaphors and you will notice they are all directed to the here and now. 'This' can refer to the present room, I think, although some participants have written responses based on the memory of say, a bedroom. This doesn't invalidate what they write, it merely suggests where their preoccupations lie. The key to the exercise, again, is the last section. 'Now, I think' seems like a safe topic, until one meets 'Now, I feel'. By dividing up thinking and feeling the emphasis falls on the last, and the participant is asked to look very directly at what is being felt, now. I can usually feel the tension building up very markedly when I ask the last three questions in this group exercise. Getting people to say things about their being and their emotions can be very frightening to them.

Discussion time after such an exercise is vital.

If you are working alone, you will want to take the time to consider whether or not you felt yourself becoming tense towards the end of the exercise, and what issues your answers may have raised. You will need to make time to write about them.

Here is another exercise in a similar vein that is designed to elicit a similar series of responses. It too is a sentence completion exercise and ideally should be used after the exercise just mentioned. This activity exists as a series of paired sentences for completion. As before, I usually read them out to a group so that there can be no prepared answers. If you are working alone with this book you may wish to place a piece of paper over the statements and move it down only as you are ready to move ahead. This prevents the eye from skipping ahead.

I like_____

But, I really like_____
_____

I hate_____

But, I really hate_____
_____

I see_____

But, I'd like to see_____
_____

I expected_____

But, I found_____

_____

I used to_____

But, now_____

_____

I pretend_____

But, now_____

_____

Take a look at the answers. I call this a double-barreled activity, because it allows us to have two shots at the same target, with a better chance
of a direct hit on the second shot. So, for example, 'I like ice cream' is almost meaningless, while 'But, I really like eating ice cream while sitting in
bed with my lover, watching t.v.' can tell a whole intimate story which
seems to link several aspects of pleasure and sexuality. Each response has
this possibility. It is only when one reaches the last two, 'I used to...' and 'I
pretend...' that the discussion moves towards aspects of behavior that were,
or may still be, unsatisfactory. 'I used to' looks back to the past, which, because it is followed by 'but now' appears to be relatively safe. It is about
something one used to do but no longer does. It is a place to discuss habits
that have been overcome, personal victories. It can also be a place to mention deepening personal failings. Compare these two responses: "I used to
eat junk food, but now I eat healthy food." and "I used to smoke cigarettes,
but now I use recreational drugs." These two responses (which actually
appeared in one session) immediately signal areas for examination. The
first person may have issues of body image and weight, or even eating disorders. The second example begs to be asked about. The individual's pain
is there for all to see. If you are working on your own the mere fact of
having written your responses down may have produced results that surprised you, as you read them over.

When we reach 'I pretend' we are in the present tense, and asking very
directly if you are willing to admit to pretenses and defenses. The 'but now'
section, therefore, can be an invitation to leave those defenses behind. One

woman wrote: "I pretend to be more confident than I am, but now I guess I'll have to stop pretending that around you folks." Of all these sentences only 'I pretend' actually confronts us, now. Each of the other sentences, just as in the first exercise in this chapter, can be responded to in a banal, concrete, fashion. One can always choose with these exercises, and that is vital, I believe, since it should not feel coercive to anyone doing these exercises. It is possible to write: "I like ice cream, but I really like it with sprinkles on top; I hate traffic but I really hate rush hour traffic; I see people in a room, but I'd like to see my friends Bill and Sue..." Even with such a bland series of responses, (and this is an actual response) it is possible to probe further. Why does this person choose traffic to hate? What can we learn about the person's life? Does this reflect any feelings about commuting to work, to school, to the group? Naturally it does. And what about 'Bill and Sue?' Is the person lonely? What is that person's sense of meaningful friendship? Even poor answers are not necessarily barren, since they may be impoverished only because the person making them is defending against the feelings that lie behind them.

In asking what any person *likes* we are asking about that person's loves, certainly about enthusiasms, and possibly about sexuality. Who could deny the sensual and sexual suggestion implicit in the licking of ice cream, after all? In talking of hate one is often talking about aspects of the self, also. It has been said that one can only truly hate what one has loved, and that one hates in others those aspects of oneself that one cannot deal with yet. I can't hate someone I do not know, but I can hate someone who has betrayed me, or cheated me, or taken unfair advantage of my help. I also know that I hate those things in others which I personally have not managed to come to terms with in myself. I hate pettiness in others, and yet I know I can be very petty when the occasion arises.

When the sentence asks about seeing 'I see...' the exercise moves into the present situation - or it can do. It can be a moment for the group to look at itself and voice expectations for themselves. It can also be a moment when participants can express their reluctance to be where they are, in the group setting. It's a good chance to spell out those feelings and acknowledge them. Indirectly this leads to the next question, about expectations and whether or not they are being met, or negative expectations (fears) and whether they are being calmed. So, one person chose to write, "I expected to be bored, but I found myself interested more than I could have hoped". Another participant was less than thrilled: "I expected detailed analysis, but I found I was expected to work at this." In each case important feelings about the present experience were raised, and needed to be discussed and recognized.

It is always possible to respond by giving past examples. Some people seem almost incapable, at first, of responding to these exercises by writing about what *is*, now. These people tend to produce memories. "I expected a train set that Christmas, but found a pad and colored pencils instead." The memory is important, of course. What does it say about the family if the child's expectation was thwarted? Did they want the child to be an artist, for example? These are important topics. But let us not forget that for such a person these historical battles and struggles are *still going on*. That is a point that needs to be introduced gently. The baggage of the past seems to have prevented the individual's concerned from living, fully, in the present.

These exercises can, I think you will agree, touch upon some very important issues within individuals. They can be used several times, of course, on the same person, so don't feel that once you have 'done' the exercise it can be of no further use. Examine what you wrote, think about it, write about it. Did you feel tense at any point? When? Why do you think that was?

Keep writing...

If we wish to take this exercise even a little further, it is possible to consider some other sentence completion exercises. Some of these may be familiar to you. I've been using these for several years, but I recently came across one of them in a book by Marcia Yudkin, and she reports good results from them also. The techniques have been in existence for a long time, I know, and variations also exist. So, with a nod to Ms. Yudkin, here is my version of the same exercise.

Take a piece of paper and ask yourself to complete the sentence "I remember". Write down your response. Then complete the sentence "I don't remember". Now repeat it four or five times in that order. Your page will look like this:

I remember_____   I don't remember _____
        _____   _____
        _____   _____
        _____   _____

Now, do the same thing again, using "I forget":

I forget   _____   I'd like to forget   _____
                  _____   _____
                  _____   _____
                  _____   _____

By now, the purpose of this exercise may be very clear to you. It is designed to get you to probe back into your personal history, and to do so indirectly. If I had asked you merely to write about your childhood, you might very well have wondered where to begin, and how to start. By asking you at first to remember and then consider what you do *not* remember I am asking you to look beyond ordinary memory to those items that may be repressed or denied. One young man wrote, "I don't remember what happened to Grandpa." He had blanked out the circumstances of his Grandfather's death, and on further investigation revealed he had been powerfully attached to the kindly old man, and felt deserted by him when he died. Until he did the exercise, however, he had not been fully aware of the strength of his attachment, nor of the powerful feelings of loss.

The sentences beginning, 'I forget...' are usually full of pleasant and less than vital information; "I forget people's birthdays/appointments/to return library books..." and so on. It is only when the question is upended to 'I'd like to forget' that one is obliged to write down what he or she has tried unsuccessfully to repress fully. It is at this point that, when working with groups, a change can occur. Group members are often very reluctant indeed to share this last series of responses. This is only natural, since the responses are likely to contain some very personal pieces of information. In normal therapeutic settings the issue of trust and confidentiality would come to the forefront and demand discussion. I would point out that for our purposes trust, although important, is not such a problem, since sharing with the group is not always vital. What is vital is that each participant should be able to spell out, on paper where it can be seen, some of the issues that are troubling him or her. As I say, in group work, it doesn't really matter if you never discuss those items with the others present, so long as you realize that these are your problems, written, identified, and indisputably there in front of you. You've identified them. You cannot pretend they do not exist. This is what you will have to look at. When you are ready you may want to talk about them, but for now it is enough to have them to think about.

If you decide that the issues you have raised are too threatening for you to tackle alone (and this is a real possibility at any stage with this book), then you should get help from a professional counselor or therapist. Do not hesitate. You will be doing the same work that you would have needed to do on yourself anyhow, but you will be doing it with a little additional support. Sometimes we all need a little private tutoring.

The whole purpose of these sentence completion exercises is to attempt to define the work that each person must acknowledge as needing to be done. No one can be forced to do that work, and that choice is the individual's personal decision. It is, however, my task to encourage you to see what areas may need to be attended to.

And that, after all, is why you're reading this book.

CHAPTER FOUR

A t this point it is probably a good idea for me to spell out a few things about what I'm trying to do with you, and why. My task is to probe through the usual conscious state and encourage you to contact the less-than-conscious state that often is so powerful in committing us to acts we barely understand. Here is an example of what I mean.

When I worked in a residential community, I noticed how, over and over again, I would reach my vacation and promptly catch the 'flu. As I lay in bed wondering why I had succumbed on the first day of vacation, again, I noticed that many of my colleagues tended to go out and make major purchases of luxury items on the same day that I traditionally fell ill. The two situations were linked, but I couldn't quite see how. On one occasion my friends came to see me and their diagnosis of me was that at the end of a tiring semester I had relaxed to such an extent that my body was no longer fighting off the germs, and so I fell ill. I was very troubled by this, as I had never thought about my 'flu bouts in this way before - always putting it down to 'bad luck'. But then I turned to one of my friends who had just purchased a stereo system he really couldn't afford, and I gave my diagnosis of his actions. "You've just given yourself a present for working hard all semester," I said. He looked at me and he was furious, then very quiet. "You're right," he said, "I don't need this stereo at all, I just wanted to have a treat."

"And you're right about my 'flu, too!" I agreed, although it took me several more weeks before I could admit it to anyone else.

I give you this example for two reasons. The first is to demonstrate how some things that 'happen' to us, like my 'flu, can often have their roots in unacknowledged actions or motivations. Just similarly the things we do to ourselves, like buying the stereo, are all products of choices we make, often without realizing why we make them. The American economy is geared toward impulse purchases, like my friend's, and often we do things without knowing why we do them, sometimes engaging thousands of dollars or major life choices in the process. Once I realized I had a pattern of getting 'flu I was, by being careful, able to moderate my behavior and not catch the virus at the end of any long or arduous piece of work. I still have to be careful, though. It was my way of falling apart only when it was safe for me to do so. My contention is that if we can find out these things, we can save ourselves a lot of time, expense, heartache and pain.

The second reason I gave you the example is quite straightforward. I could see what my friend was doing, and he could see what I was doing, but neither of us could see what we were doing to ourselves. We had to hold up the mirror to each other. If my colleagues and friends had been less open, of course, we could all have continued to be led by our unconscious motivations, in ignorance, for years. What these therapeutic writing exercises can do is help us all to hold up the mirror to ourselves. The example also teaches us a very important thing, namely that no one has to be perfect in order to offer valid advice. Our culture tends to give more credence to those with lots of letters after their names. This is not bad, naturally, but it can have the result that we tend to discredit some useful home-truths.

Often we run our lives according to our unconscious promptings, if we don't take the time to reflect. We become trapped in ways of doing things that have very little to do with what the circumstances may really demand. A woman I know who was physically abused by her mother related it in these terms. "When my first child was small I remember a specific incident. She (the child) was about two, and she accidentally knocked over her cup of milk. I knew what I could have expected from my own mother, but I found myself thinking, 'O.K. It's not necessary to hit this child.' You see, my first impulse was to repeat something that I had learned to dread as a child. Luckily I had thought about it. I didn't hit her." The conflict here was between the impulse to hit and the awareness that this reaction was not appropriate. It was only by thinking through her own experience that the woman had been able to reach the point where she didn't have to repeat her mother's abuse. It is probable that we all repeat the behavior we know unless we can see and understand reasons for changing it. It is not news to report the truism that child abusers are almost always themselves victims of child abuse, or that sexual abuse victims frequently become sexual abusers in their turn.

By exploring and understanding these barely conscious inner promptings it becomes possible to break the pattern.

If child abuse seems a somewhat extreme example possibly I should point out that there are other abuses that those who suffer can hardly understand. In my work I am constantly surprised at how common it is to come across various forms of compulsion. Over-eaters, anorexics, exercise freaks, compulsive gamblers, alcoholics, drug abusers, sex compulsives, out-of-control-shoppers, thrill junkies ... the list is endless, and the prevalence of the compulsions is staggering. Most of these unhappy people have no clear idea about why they do what they do. A few have a very clear idea about why they behave this way, and for them it is usually an avoidance of a situation, or fear, that prompts the activity. In most cases, what is unconscious is what leads the behavior.

In order to explore the meaning of the next exercise fully it will be essential to look into your childhood.

Why?

Simply, because if you understand the influences that were at work on you from those early days, you can begin to come to terms with how you got to where you are. Growing up is a little like being given directions and a road map. Where you wind up depends quite heavily on how good your directions were. That depends on who gives them to you. An example would be Estella in Charles Dickens' *Great Expectations*. The aging, embittered Miss Havisham directs Estella to break men's hearts because she was herself deserted on her wedding day. Estella, an orphan, wanting directions of any sort, follows her advice and becomes a heartless, but desperately lonely coquette.

Obviously not many people have precisely Estella's experience of life. Yet, I have worked with some women, brought up by promiscuous single mothers, who have internalized their mothers' behavior in a similar fashion. "Use men, don't trust 'em," said one, "I learned that from my Mom."

Where you wind up depends, also, on where you started.

The attitudes of our parents, or of those who brought us up, rub off on us. We accept much of who they are and many of their values, even though we may eventually reject some of those values. Those attitudes are part of the air we breathe as children, and to question them is alien to our deepest training. If we see people who have been brought up to think that people of another race are inferior, we can tut-tut, shake our heads, and wonder about the problem of racism and ignorant parenting. That is a typical reaction. If, on the other hand, we see a violent and tortured soul the chances are that we'll label that person as crazy and we will probably seek to institutionalize him or her. Please don't misunderstand. There are people who have serious mental problems that require their hospitalization and drug treatment. But there are also, as R.D. Laing pointed out, many people in hospitals whose reaction to difficult home circumstances has been to behave in such a way that they have been committed to long term care. Notice the word 'circumstances'. Some so-called mental illness is actually a rational response to a bizarre situation. One very wealthy and well-connected young man I worked with had enormous problems in his life because it seemed pointless to him to work at anything. Why should he, he argued, when he would inherit more money than he could spend? For him the 'road map' was never considered. His depression and despair, however, were very real.

These are thoughts I shall be returning to in future chapters, as we do other exercises. The exercise I want to do now is one that has been in existence for some time, and I do not know who first used it. The way in which I tend to use it, I am sure, is peculiar to me, and so if you have done something a little like this before, please do not think that this is merely a re-run of a familiar idea.

On a new sheet of paper, I would like you to draw a house that you would like to live in. Money is no object. You can draw whatever you wish, or you can draw a place that you already know, or a place you feel that could be made by adapting a place you know.

Here are some things I would like you to include in the picture, if you can, and if you wish. Put in some vegetation and some trees. Put in a door and the way one is to approach the house. You could put some scenery in, also. Is this a town house or a country house? How many windows does it have? What season of the year is it? What time of day? What's the weather doing? Which is the most important room for you? Where are the windows? Put in some sort of water as well, please, and anything else you feel you need.

This exercise will take 20 minutes or longer.

In many cases when I have done this exercise with groups, people have taken much longer, used several sheets of paper and gone to great lengths. Some have used colors, and one man wanted to make a model. Only time constraints prevented him. That will be no problem if you are working on your own with this book. Make the model, or the picture, and then read on.

Take a look at what you have drawn. Ideally someone should be on hand to ask you questions, to make you explain the picture. Few of us are such accomplished artists that we can convey our meanings without a few words to help out the drawings. Is this a house you know? A dream? Where is it? What does it convey to you - happy ideas, restful ideas, excitement? What associations does this house have for you? If you are working alone, take the time to jot down a few notes to remind yourself of these thoughts, so that you can return to this drawing months from now, if you wish, and think further.

The results of this exercise tend to fall very clearly into two categories. Some people tend to draw places they know - their relatives' houses, or a place seen and admired over a period of time. Others draw truly fantasy houses - hundreds of rooms, impossibly exotic locations, and so on. These fantasy palaces need to be seen in a different way from those places which exist in actuality, since the real houses will have memories attached to them that are often very specific. One woman drew an exact rendition of her grandmother's house (I know because she showed me a snapshot later) and explained that it was the only place she had ever been where she felt truly at peace. Any examination of the meaning of her picture would have to start from that point, I think, and the issues of parents and home-life would be the most essential topics.

The more fantastic the home, however, the more we are likely to be dealing with a symbolic representation of the psyche.

What does that mean? A house, ideally, is an expression of personality. It can say, 'I like to live like this'. Unfortunately for most of us, our bank accounts tend to dictate how we can live and one's personality is often constrained by a less than perfect house. Part of the fascination that so many people have with houses and design has to do with seeing how those with flair and money shape their houses. *Homes and Gardens*, *Country Life*, *House & Garden*, and so many other publications that sit on the magazine racks of every bookstore are evidence that the fascination is widely shared. What can compare with the excitement of seeing how Richard Gere has arranged his town house, or Sophia Loren has decorated her villa? What does it say about the personality behind the star? People flock to buy the relevant magazines.

If we accept that the house drawing you have made is a reflection of your personality, it might be useful to consider who you have portrayed yourself to be. We can make a number of blanket statements based on any picture. Like all blanket statements it is up to you to decide how far each aspect refers to you. Since I cannot see your drawing, I cannot guide you directly, I can only make suggestions.

First, look at the size of the house. Is it big or small, a hundred rooms or a log cabin in the woods? The small house may indicate a desire for coziness, seclusion, privacy. A large house tends to indicate an expansive mind that wishes to range far and wide. In Freud's writings the house was seen, in his analysis of dreams, to reflect the mind's ability to think and develop. In a famous example Freud dreamed he went into his old home and he discovered a whole room he had not known about before. This he interpreted as a message from his unconscious that he was in his professional work going into new ideas and discoveries.

Look at your drawing again. How many stories high is the house? This can tend to indicate the scope of your mental powers. Tall buildings can reflect the 'lofty thoughts' of the individual concerned. Buildings that are equipped with basements and cellars may reflect how comfortable you are with profound, deep feelings that are not easily intellectualized. One man drew a building that was three stories high, but had a vast, two level basement. He spent his whole time detailing this basement which was to contain music mixing and recording apparatus. Music, he explained, stirred him at a very profound level, allowing him to reach his deepest, emotional self. Which are you -- head in the clouds or heart in the depths of the earth? Possibly you are neither. Your house has an attic and a basement, but you choose to live on the ground floor. That is fine - it's normal because that is where we live in real life, usually. I'm merely pointing out things you may wish to consider.

Where is the door to the house? Doors can be symbols of how accessible you are, or wish to be. Many people draw fortresses when they do this exercise. Barbed wire, walls, dogs, mine fields... Not very accessible. Such people, despite what they may seem to be, are highly defensive. The door, the path or front drive, the gate and fence (if any) all these indicate how easily approachable a person is. One person had such an obstacle course for a front drive that it seemed as if one could never hope to reach the quiet log cabin on the side of a meadow. And that was the idea.

Windows, also, indicate how much one wishes to be seen, and how much one wishes to see out, to be receptive to new ideas, new influences. We call lively people in organizations by many clichés, 'a ray of sunshine', 'a breath of fresh air'. Sun and air come into stuffy rooms by way of windows, usually. The size and number of the windows can often indicate how receptive we are to outside influences.

Fireplaces, chimneys -- especially if the fire is burning -- can indicate warmth, friendliness, hospitality, food cooking, and good cheer. In the age of microwaves and central heating the fireplace has been reduced in stature, somewhat, but is still a cultural signifier, a symbol, used in movies and commercials. Liquor ads often seek to indicate the feeling of warmth and well-being the product is said to give the consumer by showing two cozy people sipping brandy next to a blazing log fire. It is one of those universal symbols that we still recognize despite the change in physical circumstances. 'The charm of a real wood stove' announced an ad in my local paper, recently. One does not get the same impression if the ad features two wholesome looking people gazing at a conventional wrought iron radiator, or a baseboard strip heater, or a thermostat switch set to 70°.

If we take the idea of fire and fireplaces further, we can suggest that as well as hospitality, food, warmth, life and the centered existence around the hearth, that it may also represent sexual warmth, and ardor. Fires in our culture have long been associated with many things, of course. Destruction, hell, anger, all these ideas have been linked to fire. But fireplaces and hearths have been seen as fire tamed, as it were, and as sexual energy. The 'fire in the blood' has indicated lusty sexual interest since before Shakespeare, and red hearts (red for lust and fire, hearts for emotions) have become a cliché of Valentine's Day. Where are the fireplaces in your drawing of the house? Are they alight? Does smoke rise from the chimneys? Again -- don't strain to find a 'meaning' to this straight away. If you haven't got any fireplaces, don't worry, it doesn't mean you're cold or asexual. One man had his house on an equatorial island paradise, so no fireplaces were needed. In this case the heat, the bodily pleasure of warmth, was all around him in his imagined home. So, use your judgments carefully, and you may learn about yourself, although you may need to mull over the ideas for a while first.

In this exercise it is always a good idea to have someone to compare
drawings with, since that can give ideas about other people's priorities. If
you are nervous about this, let me suggest another way of doing the exercise
that I discovered quite by chance. I had to take two young men, both emotionally disturbed, to the dentist on one occasion. The anxiety level was
fairly high, since cavities had to be filled, and conversation between us in
the waiting room was rather minimal. On the table were the usual well-
thumbed copies of *Reader's Digest*, *Woman's World* and so on. These were
not an attractive proposition as far as my young charges were concerned. In
amid these unappetizing magazines, however, was a copy of *The Field*, an
English magazine which, I recalled, always had excellent pictures of country
mansions in the Real Estate Sales section. I opened the magazine to a full
color advertisement of a $5 million baronial residence, and asked my com-
panions if they would pay that sort of money for that sort of house. Within
seconds we were in the most technical of discussions about what sort of
house they would have if they could, and I was learning more about their
characters than I'd believed possible. You can do the same thing with a
friend, if you wish.

Before we discuss the grounds and surrounds of the house you have
drawn, take a look at the shape of the house. Do you have any out-
buildings or wings to the house? One young man had a garage that was
easily twice the size of the house. Another man had a wing he called 'his
wing' with a special passage that connected it to the main house, through
which only he was allowed to go. A woman had placed her best friend's
house in the backyard, and another woman had a summer house for her own
private retreat. These private areas of retreat are important since they indicate a divided ego, a split between where one lives and where one does one's
private work -- be it a hobby or a job. Too emphatic a division between
these areas may indicate that the person concerned has trouble bringing his
or her whole life together, that an important part of the self does not feel it
has the chance to be expressed in the more usual living environment. Ideally, we all should be able to live whole lives in which all that we are is able
to be acknowledged by those we are close to. The novelist who does not feel
she can talk to her family about her work, but who retreats to her study, is
not connecting with them fully. The husband who feels exiled by his wife to
the workshop or the garage is in all likelihood not able to share his enthusiasms with the rest of the family. My own father had no hesitation in bringing pieces of lawnmower into the kitchen when he repaired them, claiming it

was warmer there. He was right, the temperature was warmer, and the company was always good, since that was very much the center of the house. In turn, my brother and I also used to come to the kitchen to make or repair things, until my mother became annoyed with the mess! I've noticed also how children frequently like to do their homework at the family's center. If meals are eaten at the kitchen table, that tends to become the place for homework as well. Why is this? Logically it makes more sense to work in the quiet of one's room, or even a library. Logic, of course, has nothing to do with this. These are examples of people being themselves as they work, and insisting on being themselves at the family's social center. It seems to me that it is not until the upper levels of high school or college that young people can study alone in quiet corners for any length of time. By then the subject is often so rarefied that the individual already feels like an exile, reading about a topic that is remote from everyday life. It makes perfect sense to do that away from the family. Where is your private area in your drawing?

As we look at the grounds of the house you have drawn, note the time of day and season of the year. These all have to do with the individual's mood, and sense of where he or she is in life at this moment. It can also indicate when one hopes to move to the house. One woman drew her house in the fall -- her favorite time of year because it was restful, she said. Fall tends to suggest the ending of the year, and so her attitude to herself (was she in the autumn of her life?) would be different from someone who specified spring time. In the years that I have been doing these exercises I have seen mostly summertime depicted, and usually the middle part of the day. On two occasions, only, have I had group members produce pictures with a night-time setting. One was by a woman of 70 who drew the house she had just sold, and in which her husband had recently died. The other was by a young man with a very romantic but gloomy temperament. Again, rarely has anyone presented a picture with bad weather, and only once have I received a snow scene. From this I can only guess that in this area of the U.S. (the Northeast) the usual tendency is towards summer and sunlight in those aged 18 to 65, regardless of the season of year in which the exercise is done. It may be different if you are in Alaska, of course. What is important is to see what is drawn in *relation* to what seems to be considered 'usual'. The entire process of uncovering aspects of the self is exactly like detective work, in as much as the clues are there, but few of them can be said definitely to mean something on their own. It is the totality of clues that matters.

With this in mind, let us look at the vegetation. Is the house crowded by bushes and trees? This could indicate someone who feels crowded, hemmed in. Trees can be indicative of relationships with friends. How many trees are there? How close to the house are they? Big trees, close to the house tend to reflect strong, close ties with a few people. My own picture has four trees quite close to the house, which I take to be the true reflection of my friendships -- a few, but very important. As it happens, I would agree that I have four very close friends. This interpretation is not always true for everyone, however. A woman I worked with was frightened of trees, especially big ones. She had no trouble finding friends, however. For her, this exercise would be colored by personal concerns of a different sort.

Elaborate gardens do not usually appear in the drawings I have seen. I think this has to do with the fact that most of the people I've worked with neither have big houses themselves, nor have much gardening experience with large spaces. Rolling lawns seem to appear a great deal, and horse paddocks. Dogs and cats appear also. Taking a broadly Freud and Jung based approach to these animals in the pictures, we can say that whatever they represent in personal terms ("My dog, Toby", "A horse I'd like to own one day") they also indicate the physical, instinctual side of the person who included them. The horse's strength and size, and its sexual value -- one bestrides a horse -- can indicate how the drawer feels about his or her body and sexuality. Dogs and cats are loving and love to be petted, which suggests a cozy and unthinking love willingly offered by a cuddly creature. Cats are a little more independent than most dogs, and so the preference of one or the other pet can indicate something about the type of love one feels comfortable accepting. Dogs are intensely attached to their owners. Is that the sort of love you are willing to accept from a person? That sort of dependence? Or are you a cat lover?

The last item I want to discuss here is the water feature I asked you to include. What is it? A lake? A river? The sea? One woman put a faucet in her garden with a dripping tap. A man who did this exercise had a small bird bath. A young man had a waterfall some yards from his house. What does this mean?

Water can be seen as many things. It gives life, of course, it is also seen as a primarily female symbol, one linked to the emotions and sexuality. Venus (the Goddess of Love) is depicted arising from the sea in Botticelli's *Birth of Venus*, and Poseidon, the God of the Sea, was always seen as passionate and emotional rather than rational. The water in the picture then, can indicate how one feels about one's emotional, instinctual, sexual side, the so-called 'female' side of one's self. A stagnant puddle, for example, would suggest that the life-giving values of water, its movement, its depth, its crystal clarity - all are gone. A person drawing such a pool may well be feeling that life and living are dull and irksome. Water is life. Draw a dead puddle and there can be no life. One woman, bitterly upset by her divorce and seeing no future for herself, drew such a puddle. Young men seem to like to draw lakes with motorboats and jet skis that they use to zoom across the surface. These boats usually are symbols of masculine phallic power vigorously rushing around enjoying the 'female' sexuality of the lake. The boat cutting a wake in the lake is a relatively new item, historically, but the cliché of the male plowing the Mother Earth to raise a harvest later is as old as civilization, and is a metaphor for the sexual union of male and female. A boat, likewise, plows a wake, making it a doubly sexually loaded symbol.

These are only suggestions for possible interpretations of your picture. You may feel outraged by these suggestions, in which case I have to ask you to consider the question, why are you so upset? One woman I worked with was so upset that she might have revealed something that she had not wanted to that she immediately drew another house saying, "This is the real me." I doubted that. The 'real' her probably existed somewhere between the fantasy house she was afraid to acknowledge and the anemic version she replaced it with. Sometimes the reverse happens. One young woman drew a pretty little house at first, confessed that she had wanted to draw a *much* more daring picture, but had felt afraid to do so. She then proceeded to produce a wonderfully extravagant picture, unleashing all her dreams as she did so. For her it was a major turning point, even though it was not entirely successful on the first attempt. So think about your picture. Are you comfortable with it? If you had to change something, what would it be? Remember, only change something if it is, to you, a truer representation of how you feel. Don't draw a larger lake because you wish to impress your friends with your sexual confidence. That does no one any good.

CHAPTER FIVE

All that we have done so far has fallen under the broad category of 'naming'. When you drew the house or jabberwocky you were naming, in a less conventional way, the important areas of your life that you probably would have found it hard to express any other way.

Naming is one of our most powerful coping strategies. because of this, it can often slip back upon us and leave us with just the name of the problem but no desire to alter the situation. "I'm really screwed up," announced one young man, "but I'm kind of happy with it." The only trouble was that he radiated misery and conflict. In his case identifying that a problem existed was not enough to make him move further ahead. As time went on he became more and more attached to his neurosis -- after all, he'd taken a lifetime to develop it -- and less and less inclined to change. Sometimes, for many of us, if happiness seems unobtainable, it can be a great relief at least to have an identity as being unhappy. It's better than nothing. Again, the same problem often exists with abused and battered wives. Living with an abusive spouse may well be hell, but for many women it may feel preferable to the uncertainty of life alone. The identity one has is less risky, it seems, than making a change. Better the devil you know... This simplifies the problem rather drastically, but I use it because I suspect that naming any problem can be helpful only if it is accompanied by the desire to move ahead.

All these exercises, all my words, are only of any use if you really want to move ahead.

This brings me to my next topic, which is another example of a coping strategy: rhythm.

Rhythm is built into all we do. Have you ever awakened at 9:30am having overslept? You rush to get to work, skip breakfast, forget to brush your teeth... The usual ritual of the morning has been hopelessly upset. If you're like me, it can upset the whole of the day. I feel out of phase until I can get to sleep that night. That is a simple example of the disruption of a familiar routine, and I'm sure you can add your own examples. As a college professor I know that an 8:30am class is never likely to be as scintillating as one at 11:30am, or to fill as readily with students. And I also know that the working week has its own rhythm, too. For a while, in the 1970s, one could buy cars built on a Friday at a cheaper rate than the more 'normal' cars -- since the Friday product was acknowledged to be of less high quality. Workers would be tired and anxious to go home, it was argued, and so do a less good job of assembly.

Factory work, interestingly enough, is built upon rhythms. The famous British tea-break was not provided simply because tender-hearted employers felt the workers needed a cup of hot tea. It was instituted in munitions factories during the First World War simply because it was found to be more efficient. At the start of hostilities workers had labored until they fell asleep at the machines. The loss of time and money caused by accidents and incorrectly assembled pieces made the employers realize that an enforced break and a limit on overtime actually made for higher production and higher quality. Merely forcing people to work flat out, beyond their need for food and sleep, was self-defeating. Again, the assembly line today is carefully designed to move along at a certain speed. This speed has been determined, usually, by negotiations between employers, the employees' unions, and time and motion experts. Run the conveyor belt too fast and the job cannot be done properly; run it too slowly and the workers become bored and so fail to do the work properly. Run the conveyor at varied unpredictable speeds and the workers become very upset indeed!

What is astonishing, here, is that speeds can be set fairly accurately that suit most workers. Human beings appear to exist at very similar levels of rhythms. Yet these rhythms are also very individual. A straightforward example is if you have ever shared a home with someone who does not like to get up and go to bed at the same time as you do, or who eats according to a different schedule. Or try flying across the Atlantic and notice how out of phase you are with the rhythms of the day in the place at which you arrive.

In rural England, where I grew up, restaurants opened at lunch time from 11:30am to 1:30pm, after which time no hot food was available. In the evening they would open at 6:00pm and stop serving food at 9:00pm, often earlier. Friends of mine who arrived from America could hardly believe that they couldn't get a hot meal at certain times of the day. Yet the local population had all fitted in to the local rhythm.

These days we call these biorhythms. Strictly speaking, a biorhythm is one's internal body rhythm, but we learn other rhythms from our surroundings -- such as the meal-time rhythm. And, just as an aside, notice how some people become anxious and grumpy if they don't eat regularly or on schedule. Their internal clock is telling them to eat, now. As a general rule, it is not easy to work with people in this state since they are literally not themselves. I think, however, that it is well worth looking deeper than this.

In a now famous experiment, some coastal oysters were moved into the center of the United States, in special tanks. No one understood how the oysters knew when to open their shells in order to catch the nutrients carried to them by the tidal flow. How did they know the tide was about to turn? The rationale behind the experiment was that if the shellfish were moved a long way from the sea and placed in calm water, how they coped with the change would reveal how they functioned. Were their actions learned behavior, or genetically programmed? After the shellfish had settled down, they all developed the same rhythm of opening and closing. Further investigation revealed that they were opening at exactly the same time the tide would have been coming in if there had been a tide in the middle of the U.S. But how had they been able to calculate this? The question was pondered deeply and the solution was surprising. The humble shellfish were responding to the gravitational pull of the moon, which is what causes the tides to flow around the globe.

So what does this have to do with us? I would suggest that if the shellfish of the world respond to the moon, then we human beings, who are over 90% water, are probably similarly affected, but we tend not to know or notice because we're too involved in our daily activities. Ask anyone who has ever worked in a long term psychiatric ward -- the time of the full moon is often a time of some unrest. Lunatic, itself, is a term derived from the Latin word 'luna', the moon, because madmen were often seen to be at their most active at the time of the full moon. Every woman knows that she menstruates, on average, every 28 days, and this too is thought to be tied in to the lunar calendar. More curious still is the frequently-observed phenomenon that women living in close proximity find that their menstrual cycles have coincided exactly, through no obvious volition of their own. The 'rhythm method' of birth control is also tied in directly to the ovulation and menstruation rhythms of women, and couples who wish to avoid conception can calculate (with the help of temperature charts and calendars) exactly when the woman is likely to be her most receptive, and plan accordingly. The same process works the other way for couples who are anxious to have children or have found conception difficult.

None of this should come as any surprise to us. A baby in the womb becomes aware of the heart beat of its mother, and if one wishes to comfort the new child, every mother knows that by placing him or her against her chest, where the child can hear the mother's heart, the baby is reassured. Just similarly rhythmic rocking, stroking, or singing can placate children. The old trick of comforting a new puppy by wrapping a loudly ticking alarm clock in flannel works the same way. The puppy tends to think the sound is its mother's heartbeat, and sleeps in peaceful deluded assurance. At least, that's what we think the puppy thinks!

I'm sure you can provide your own examples of rhythm and how it works, but I'll give you a few more examples because I think they are important. When I worked with autistic children I became rapidly aware how comforting they found the structure of the day. Any diversion from the usual structure could upset them very badly. I also noticed that when we were in the playground that it was extraordinarily difficult to get those children to leave the swings. The to and fro movement caused them to smile beatifically, and I do believe they would have swung all day had they been allowed to. Some of the children also had other rhythmic preoccupations; some rocked on their chairs, some scratched or rubbed repeatedly, others had to have padded headgear to prevent them from banging their heads over and over again. Joost Meerloo (in Jack Leedy's *Poetry Therapy*, 1969) has suggested that for these children the rhythmic motion is so comforting that even extreme action like head banging or rectal digging becomes preferable to the unpredictable outside world. If we look at these children as similar to ourselves in some ways, we can argue that rhythm, or the imposing of rhythm, is a primary defense that allows a chaotic world to be perceived as orderly. J.H. Masserman has suggested this much.

I would tend to agree. We talk of people being 'out of synch' with each other. North Americans traveling in southern American countries often tell tales of being frustrated to the point of madness by the relaxed attitude of those from the warmer corners of the continent, and the fact that trains, planes, and buses do not run on time - where 'on time' is their own version of the phrase. Another example is that it can be very stressful to talk with someone who always interrupts, or who speaks fast and will not allow us to say anything. Such a person is literally living at a different speed from ourselves, and we are unlikely to be able to feel relaxed with such a companion. I can usually tell if I'm going to like someone by the way the rhythm of conversation develops. There should be, for me, give, then take, then give...and so on. With this in mind, it is worth noting that one of the most devastating and powerful forms of torture that has been used in questioning suspects is not the application of direct pain. Instead it has been described as sensory deprivation. The victim is not allowed to know what time it is, what day it is, where he or she is, or what is going to happen. Artificial light only is used, (sometimes total darkness is imposed by way of variation) and there are no outside views. Food arrives irregularly, is bland, and the victim no longer knows if he or she is getting hungry at the 'right' time. Sleep is disrupted, cells are changed frequently for no reason, and all cells are kept similarly drab. Faced with this ghastly situation, with all familiar sights gone, and no sense of time, ten minutes can seem like hours, and a few days like an eternity. The victim's sense of self quickly collapses.

We love rhythm and structure. Without it we become distressed. The unemployed man or woman can easily get side tracked from the rhythm of work and looking for it, and in no time at all we can see the alert salesclerk becoming a wistful figure, unwashed, eating junk food, still in a bathrobe at 4:00 pm -- rudderless. The converse example would be the executive on vacation, who cannot relax because he or she is still on the work schedule. I am convinced that part of the appeal of Hitler's Nazis and Mussolini's Fascisti lay in the rigid order they imposed on two national economies that were in chaos. From chaos to order -- even order such as they offered -- was a very attractive move for many voters. Each party, interestingly enough, loved rhythmic marching, chanting and salutes. One has only to watch archive footage of the crowds chanting 'Seig Heil' (pronounced *Seeg Hìle*) or 'Duce' (pronounced *Doo-chày*) to realize that the quick one-two rhythm of the cry had an almost mesmeric quality for many. Why does that matter? Well, the same technique of hypnotic jingles that misled an entire culture, causing massive destruction and death -- a variation of that same technique is used today in advertising. I can remember jingles I heard when I was 8, for products I never used. The rhythms stuck in my brain, all those years, no matter whether I wanted them there or not. The Pepsodent ad remains alongside W.B. Yeats and T.S. Eliot in my memory. Perfect poetry, rhythmically pleasing, and used for entirely different reasons. Those Nazis knew *exactly* what they were up to.

To return to rhythm in its present form, we have only to gaze at the monuments of the past. Stonehenge, whatever else it may be said to be, certainly *is* a solar calendar. The Nazca lines in Peru, which stretch for miles across the desert, are also calendars, and so are many of the European standing stones and stone circles. In a pre-literate culture, it was vitally important to know when to plant crops and harvest them. In a climate like that of Northern Europe with mild winters and no extremes of temperature, it would have been difficult for farmers to know with any precision what time of year it was, and to plan accordingly. When should the bull be placed with the cows? The ram with the sheep? Accurate calendar work was vital for success, and so, in a real sense, it gave order to chaos.

I have written about this at some length because I believe it is a very important topic. Rhythm enters all we do. As I said earlier in the book, in group work it is often very important to start on time and end on time, since stress can be generated all too easily if members feel that a session is open ended. Similarly, members become primed for the sessions in advance, ready to raise issues at that once-a-week or twice-a-week meeting. If the meetings are random, then it is difficult to get members to be ready on time, and so the whole process becomes much more fraught with anxiety.

That is why I have arranged this book as I have. Each chapter has a beginning preamble before we get to the exercises. I have done this quite consciously. In group work, I find that this structure (of me giving information and then moving to an exercise) lasts about six weeks. By that time, I find that group members are bringing in their own ideas and preoccupations in the first half, and my informational preambles tend to be relegated to the sidelines. I deliberately set up a structure so that the revealing and often anxiety-producing exercises are placed at a recognizable time, and this rhythm helps participants to stay calm and to respond more fully when the exercise does occur.

For the person who is working with this book alone, rhythm can be immensely helpful. Try setting aside a certain portion of the day, or part of one day a week, when you will read this book and do the exercises. Ideally you should establish a schedule that will allow you to do the exercises and then, a certain amount of time later, give yourself the space to review what you did and write some more. This works very well for some people. They discover that they have internalized the schedule to the point at which they sit at their desks, prepared to write, and discover that the thoughts and ideas are positively bursting from them. Just as our bodies know to get hungry at lunchtime, despite anything we may tell our stomachs, so our minds can be trained to look inward at certain times.

There is always a drawback, though. Despite the fact that I have at-tempted to use a consoling rhythm in the application of these exercises, we will have to be aware that rhythms can cause us to become stuck. Rhythms do comfort us, often to the extent that we stay in the reassuring repetition of a hum-drum existence, sometimes for years. Locked in our own little world we can forget the passing of our lives all too easily. Rhythm may give shape and meaning to the day, but it can also deaden the responses. This is the double-edged sword we have at our disposal, and it appears over and over again.

Rhythm can shape our day -- and dull our world.

Naming can help us see a problem -- and stop us getting any further. ("I gotta learning disability" announced one young man, "You can't expect me to do anything." With an I.Q. of 150, I did expect something from him, and eventually he made progress.)

Forgetting, or 'denial' as it is known, provides the same double-edge. It can help us cope with the pain of the past -- and can also stop us dealing with the damage that came with the pain., ("I don't have a drinking problem except when I can't get a drink", declared a Tee-shirt. Who are they fool-ing?)

The very strengths our minds possess can often work against us, and that is one reason for these exercises, since we attempt to by-pass the usual methods of inquiry and take ourselves by surprise. Find a sheet of paper. I would like you to think of something that happened to you in your life that you felt you had to apologize for, even though you meant whatever it was at the time. Write a bogus apology -- you can be as sarcastic and as irreverent as you wish. Write several.

This exercise takes some 20 minutes, usually, for the writing and quite a lot longer for the sharing of apologies. What will emerge here is anger about a variety of items. Some are day-to-day, but all have to so with deeper tendencies. The person who writes with hilarity about yelling at another driver on the road may well be angry about commuting such a long distance to work. What lies behind this? Is the home situation not ideal, causing the person to have to drive long distances because of the needs of spouse or children to live in that particular place?

The repressed anger of the day can be expressed in these bogus apologies. That alone can be healthy. It's known by some as 'venting' -- just getting it off one's chest. That is the first level.

The second level that emerges, if you are with others in a group, is the recognition that one gains that one is not alone in feeling this way. "Wow!" exclaimed one young man, "I thought I was the only person who yelled at other drivers. Now I see you're all doing it, I don't feel so bad."

The third level is where we attempt to find the anxiety or upset behind the initial anger. The man who abuses another driver may have just had an argument with his spouse or his boss, and the issues in those arguments may be profound indeed. Thwarted dreams, a sense of being undervalued, despair -- all these can lurk behind the 'bogus apology'. If, in group work, the individual can reach this third level and express it, we are suddenly at the fourth level. Level four is the point at which, through sharing, the group members realize that the topics they have raised are very important, profoundly so, and they are often astonished that they can talk openly in front of comparative strangers. They take themselves seriously, at this point, and regard others the same way. In doing this the entire therapeutic process, all these exercises, all this talk -- the entire thing is revalued.

If you are working on your own, it may be hard to understand this. Let me put it another way. This exercise was specifically designed to find out what you are angry about. Now, suppose I had simply asked: What are you angry about? The chances are very good that almost no one would have admitted to being angry. Result -- nothing. No anger here, thank you. The truth of the matter is that we are, often, very angry and many times we don't know it. When I do this exercise, I am always interested to see how many people write bogus apologies to girl/boyfriends not seen for a long time. I've written many such myself, about a relationship that ended years ago. The truth is that I was still angry at this person -- and at myself for being such a fool. This is not merely an unhealthy re-run of emotions that have no need to be resurrected. Personally, I know that relationship was a major error in my life, but luckily one I could learn from. By reminding myself of this I consider that I reduce the chances of slipping into another relationship like it. And that is healthy!

And that is the whole secret of the bogus apology. It does not just tap into our anger. It shows us our anger and the fact that we can learn from it if we want to. The 'apology' is a way of admitting that we ourselves are partly to blame, and that we are not going to repeat the error. Here are some examples:

"I'm sorry that you feel you have to leave me after all this time, but I can see your point. After all, you've spent all my money, so why should you stay?"

"Forgive me. I dented your car. After all the time you spent working on it and waxing it when you could have been talking with me..."

"I'm really sorry I answered back and told you what I really think about the way you live and the way you've treated me. I shouldn't expect much, right? You must be so used to walking all over my needs..."

Notice the way the anger *includes* the fact that the speaker had some part in what went wrong. It is only when we can admit our part in our own problems that we can hope to change things. If it is always a case of 'them' doing something to us, we cast ourselves in the role of helpless victim. Nothing can change if one is helpless.

Here is an example from Aeschylus' *Oresteia* that may help to show what I mean. The Greek dramatists often conveyed extremely subtle insights in their works. That is probably why the plays have survived in such high regard for so long. In my experience literature that is short on human value rarely lasts two decades, let alone two millennia. Orestes, the hero of this drama, has a dreadful problem, He has to kill his father's murderer according to Greek tradition. Unfortunately, his father was killed by his mother -- who was herself avenging the death of her daughter. The father, Agamemnon, had sacrificed his daughter to the gods in return for a swift passage to Troy. His wife, Clytemnestra, was duty-bound to kill him as a result. Now, Orestes is stuck with a duty he realizes is a terrible thing to do. (Hamlet had a similar problem, in some ways). Orestes kills his mother and for his evil deed is tortured by the Furies, who drive him almost mad. Tormented, Orestes petitions the gods, arguing that since he had no choice in the matter he cannot be held accountable. The gods convene and hold a trial. Apollo argues convincingly for Orestes, and just as they are about to pardon Orestes, he stops the proceedings, declaring that it was he, not the gods, who killed his mother.

The moment he admits he has played a part in this disaster, a miracle occurs. The Furies leave him, and instead he is visited by the muses - the spirits of music, poetry, dance, art, and so on.

The human value of the episode should not elude us. If we admit our errors, the pain can be converted into creative energy and wisdom. Don't we owe it to ourselves to get to that point?

Another exercise that works approximately the same way is this. I call it the silly diary entry. We've all had the experience of sitting down to write to a friend to whom we owe a letter and ... nothing in our lives seems interesting enough to write about. Or we take out our journals, saying, 'I really must write something this week,' and our minds go blank. Only trivia remains. Woke up, went to work, came home, slept. That sort of thing. Well now is your big chance. Write an outrageous, silly, bizarre journal entry.

This exercise needs about 20 minutes for the writing and usually provides enough material for about an hour's discussion.

The results are usually hilarious or at the very least, strange. One young woman who was very fitness-conscious described being kidnapped by aliens and being forced to eat candy bars, none of which made her fat, luckily. As the discussion proceeded she revealed that she is obsessive about food and exercise, that she loves candy but does not allow herself to eat any. Behind her revelation, however, lay a profound unease about food. This in turn allowed two other women (both former bulimics) to offer her their support and understanding, which she, herself, found it a little difficult to accept.

One young man described a hilarious party with his father dancing with all the young women and throwing empty beer cans at a police cruiser, being arrested and wisecracking with the judge. It turned out that the father was an almost entirely silent man, addicted to t.v. and very dull company indeed. The young man himself loved to party and had very recently nearly been arrested after a drinking spree. The discussion that followed led him to consider what he wanted from his relationship with his father, and whether he was attempting to make his partying some sort of substitute for his estrangement from his father.

A woman wrote about meeting Robert Redford in her local supermarket and advising him how to pick out the ripe peaches, while her five- and seven-year-old children stood beside her discussing Tolstoy. This allowed her to talk, later, about how dull her life was, and how much work the children could be. Her gentle fantasy of flirtation -- the oblique sexuality of squeezing ripe fruit made her giggle -- and of her children becoming verbal rather than merely noisy, caused her much laughter. It enabled her to see that her situation really was dull, and that she craved both physical affection and mental stimulation (talk about Tolstoy and literature). As she laughed at the absurdity she was able to acknowledge that Robert Redford never would walk into her local suburban supermarket, and that it would be some time before her small children could meet her intellectual needs. And here's the important part: in each case the acknowledgment that the individuals who appeared in the fantasies could not fulfill the need meant that the expectation changed. The woman found she could accept that her kids were merely normal five- and seven-year-olds. Instead of resenting what they could not provide, which she craved, she simply accepted that she'd have to get her mental stimulation elsewhere. The resentment and anger towards them faded. The young man also, instead of being angry at his father for being a couch-potato, recognized he'd never get much action from him and should not resent him for not measuring up to the needs the son felt.

This exercise used a reversal, as most of the others have. The reversal was simply in not asking what the situation is, but what it is not. The house exercise, you may remember, did not ask you to write about who you are and want to be, but to draw the place you want to live in. The jabberwock drawing did not require you to write and talk about a fear but to draw something that could be fearsome. The last exercise we did returns to the idea of rhythm. Some times the daily rhythm can dull us to what is really happening. That is the negative side of rhythm, making us overlook important things. The conveyor belt system is not only efficient, it is also vaguely anesthetic, causing the worker not to think too much. This exercise seeks to reclaim that which is obliterated by custom.

Use this information. Write about the things you tend to take for granted because of the way your day is arranged. Imagine what it would be like if one key element of the day changed. What if there was a transportation strike? What if your car died? Try to remember what it was like when these things happened in the past. What did you do the day the snowstorm meant you couldn't go to work? Change the rhythm and see what you learn.

CHAPTER SIX

In the previous section we talked about things that we overlook, ignore and repress. We all do this, and it is healthy, for the most part. We overlook the faults of a loved one because we are concentrating on the things we love, and the annoying personal habits are ignored. Sometimes we find ourselves doing that to a degree that is unhealthy. We pretend someone in our family does not have a substance abuse problem -- for whatever reasons we pretend. This is known as denial.

Denial comes in various forms. A man I know told me, "When I was 17 I got a girl pregnant. Her folks were rich and cared about their reputation in the town, so they paid for an abortion. They called my parents and my folks looked at me sternly and said, "We're never going to talk about this again." At 17 I couldn't believe my ears. I'd done this thing and everyone was pretending it hadn't happened. But I knew it had. It was the worst thing I'd ever done in my life and I wasn't even getting a slap on the wrist." This is very conscious denial -- an arranged conspiracy not to say anything.

Another example that I came across was within a family. The aging and senile grandfather had developed a habit of grabbing his genitals and rubbing energetically whenever a woman was present in the room. Otherwise he was fairly normal. His niece, who was the one who was most perturbed by this, called a family meeting and asked what was to be done about this problem, since the hired nurses who were to look after the old man kept quitting in protest. Every single other member of the family, all of whom had seen this strange behavior for themselves, immediately denied that the grandfather had any behavioral quirks at all. Most denial is not as obvious as this. It is much more low key. We tend to forget the mean-spirited things we have done, for instance; we have another slice of chocolate cake and say that we'll start that diet 'tomorrow'.

How denial and repression work is open to question, and in order to understand it, we will have to look at different theories about how the mind works. Freud, in a by now famous statement, said that memory and consciousness are often at war. "My memory says, 'I did this'; my mind says, 'That cannot be so'. The mind usually wins." In severe cases the person concerned may blot out a memory completely - no recollection may remain at all of a catastrophic event. Sexual abuse, violence, deaths of loved ones, all can be blotted out by this defensive amnesia, at least for a while. This is *repression*. It is a way of dealing with a difficult circumstance in the short term. If the circumstance is not given space to be acknowledged it will tend to surface again later. If you need a comparison, repression is like an aspirin. It dulls the pain in the short term. It is not a cure for the reason the pain is there in the first place. One can deaden toothache by taking aspirin, but eventually the gum becomes infected if the tooth is not dealt with. If one pretends then that the gum is not in a dangerous condition, that is *denial*. So the short-term fix can lead to the long-term problem, since denial usually manifests itself in dangerous behavior of some sort. Alcohol abuse and drug abuse frequently are ways of getting "out of one's head" because what is inside the head has not been acknowledged and dealt with. 'I drink to forget' is a cliché of the comic strip bar-fly, but if one has disturbing memories alcohol will not cause them to disappear. It will merely damage the liver and cause hangovers.

This leads us into a discussion of how the mind works. There are many theories, and since none can be proved, they remain theories. Some, I think, are better than others, but all are useful if we wish to understand ourselves. What follows, here, are shamelessly brief assessments of some theories, given my own particular bias. If any of these appeal to you, you may want to read further, and the reading list at the end of the book is for just that reason.

Freud suggested the mind is made up of three main elements. The Id, the Ego and the Superego. These are arranged as follows:

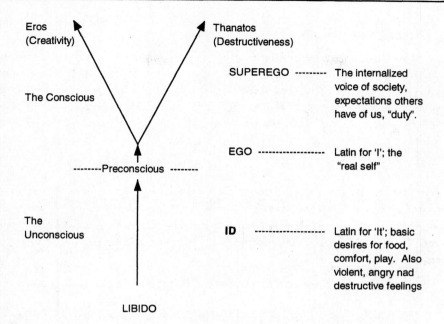

The theory is that we start life at the Id level, as babies, and that we are a bundle of undisciplined wants. Gradually the world imposes its expectations upon us, and we internalize those as the Superego. We do not always do those things that we want, but those things that authority figures tell us we should do. We save money sensibly rather than spending it all the moment we have it.

Gradually the Ego emerges. The Ego is the part that is our individuality. The Id says, 'Spend all the money, *now*.' The Superego says, 'Save it' and the Ego decides to spend some now and save some for later. Each person develops his or her own value systems as the Ego develops. We find that we don't always believe all that authorities tell us. Norman Holland in *Poems in Persons* (Norton, 1975) suggests that the Ego is constantly mediating between the Superego and the Id and that it constantly attempts to find new ways of balancing them. That is a person's individual style, he suggests, and the diagram Freud gave us is amended to look like this

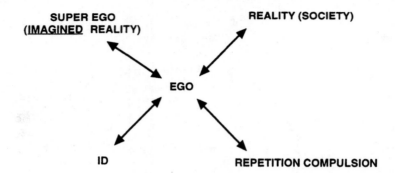

The Ego has to do a lot of work in all this to let us know who we are.

Freud has more to say about this. He suggested that the Id dwells in the unconscious part of ourselves, and that the Libido emerged from there, also.

The Unconscious is that part of ourselves that we are vaguely aware of. It is what makes us prefer a Corvette to a Hyundai or spaghetti to curry, or whatever.

The Libido can be defined as sexual energy. Sexual energy, according to Freud, was the main driving force behind human actions, and it could be directed two ways. The first, obvious way, is towards sex and the production of children. This Freud calls the Eros urge, named after the Greek god of love and from which we get the word erotic. The urge can go any number of different ways, as it happens. Sexuality itself was, to Freud, polymorphous, which meant that like an explosion it would go wherever it could, or wanted to. There is no 'right' way for sexuality to go because where it goes might depend upon what opportunities it may have. In the absence of women, men may develop sexual relationships with each other or simply prefer their own sex even if women are present. It is only society that pressures us to what it considers 'normal' behavior. The libido is under pressure, and sometimes it does not turn to procreation as an outlet. The person who decides to build empires or monuments to his or her own greatness is fulfilling the same urge to leave a creation that will live on, just as the parent leaves children who will perpetuate the family line. This desire to memorialize the self Freud called the Thanatos instinct, named after the Phoenician goddess of death. These are Yeats' 'monuments of unaging intellect'. Our civilization is filled with examples of those who traded in family coziness and fulfillment for fame and recognition. An example would be the businessman who is so busy working to leave a fortune to his family that he never sees his wife and children. For whatever reasons he finds it easier to deal with business than real people in an intimate atmosphere. Another example might be the film star who is so glamorous on screen and whose life is filled with personal pain. These examples are still borderline, since the most obvious use of the Thanatos instinct is the aggressive drive to make war and perpetuate one's memory through conquest. The sexual energy has been completely inverted.

Freud's idea of Superego, Ego and Id has gained wide acceptance in our time. It is the basis of the recent idea that within each of us there are three people; the child, the adult, and the parent. The phrases 'inner child' and 'inner adult' are popular buzz words today, and have been so widely adopted that it would be unfair to attribute any one person with their existence. The only disadvantage of the idea as far as I can tell, is that if we allow three inner figures, what is to prevent us from allowing more? What about the 'inner lover' or the 'inner delinquent'? Possibly it is unfair to ask those questions, since all that any theory can do is to offer a framework or a language that can be used to help us reassess a confusing phenomenon. Theories are ways of naming, too.

Professor Marie Murphy has recently made me aware of some interesting information that has become available about the way the human brain grows. Briefly stated it seems that the brain exists in three sections, moving from the spinal cord towards the front of the head. The 'primitive' brain, nearest the spinal column, controls basic bodily functions that are involuntary. Breathing, digestion, reflex actions and so on are centered here. Children are born with this part of the brain well developed, and as they grow the section of the brain ahead of this begins to grow too. This new section deals with motor skills, language acquisition, memory, and sensory processing. All the skills a growing school child needs to master. It is not until puberty that the brain begins to grow again, this time in the frontal areas. These frontal lobes would seem to be responsible for moral and ethical speculation, theoretical concerns which involve areas of doubt and conjecture. This gives a new slant to the Superego, Ego and Id triad.

C.G. Jung, Freud's pupil and friend who later argued bitterly with him, developed a slightly different series of ideas. He produced several different diagrams of the psyche in an attempt to clarify his thoughts. His most readily accepted idea is that of Introvert and Extrovert personalities. One is either inward looking (Introverted) or outward (Extroverted) in the way one presents oneself. Within this he put forward the idea of the 'compass' of the psyche which looks like this:

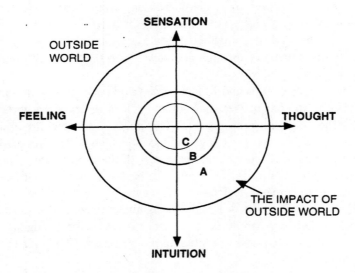

REGION A -   THE CONSCIOUS MIND, WHICH DEALS WITH THE
              OUTSIDE WORLD

REGION B -   THE UNCONSCIOUS

REGION C -   THE COLLECTIVE UNCONSCIOUS, WHICH HOLDS
              THE MEMORIES OF ALL HUMANITY, AND CONTAINS
              THE ROOTS OF THE FOUR FUNCTIONS: FEELING,
              THOUGHT, INTUITION, SENSATION

The four elements are opposed -- a person who lives on feelings is likely to be less involved in detached rational thinking, and a person who responds to intuition is going to look past the world of the senses. We all have each of the elements, but all of us have a slightly different balance.

Jung then drew his own chart of the layers of the psyche. It looks like this:

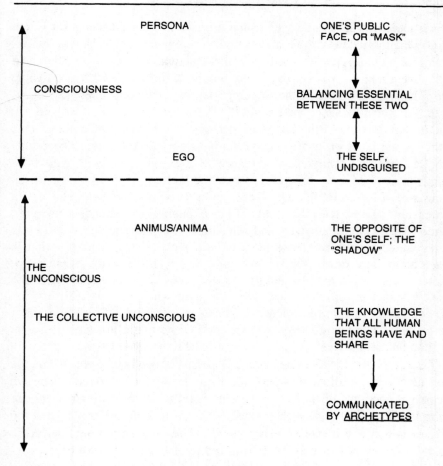

Jung maintained that our collective unconscious is always trying to communicate with our conscious selves, and that it is a sort of tribal wisdom into which we tap when we choose to recognize it. Mankind should attempt to make that contact, according to Jung, but unfortunately most of us exist at the level of social activity, or Persona, and never bother to look elsewhere for who we are.

If all this seems very confusing, I would wish to reassure you here. Freud's and Jung's diagrams of the psyche are basically very similar. Each has four levels. Notice Freud's Libido comes from some un-named region well below the Id; giving us a 4th level. What this means for us is that there is an underlying emphasis in each diagram that there are levels of existence.

This is exactly what I have been trying to show whenever I mention the levels at which any deed can be understood. For example: you draw a house. Everyone would agree it is a house and that within certain boundaries it looks like a house. It is not the size of an apple, for instance. It is a livable size. This corresponds to the Superego layer, since our Superegos recognized the socially sanctioned request to draw a house, and we did so. Within that drawing of the house are personal, individual preferences. This is the second layer of awareness, which is to do with the Ego. The details may be fantastic or playful. The man who drew a fortress with guns bristling from it was hardly producing a realistic house. He was expressing his own sense of his desire to be protected and secure in a fortress. This desire came from the next level down, the Id layer roughly corresponding to Jung's 'shadow self'. The man who had felt vulnerable and frail as a child has compensated royally for those fears he *still feels*. That is partly what is meant by the idea of the 'shadow'. This is the part of the self that is the opposite of who we seem to be and this aspect needs always to be brought into contact with the conscious self. So, the man who drew the fortress felt fragile; what he chose to project was the exact opposite. If he could admit the feelings of vulnerability which are internal he might not have to waste his time on the massive structures of external defense.

The fourth level is that level which is almost beyond our grasp -- it is the level at which we all exist, where we all have similar behavior, where we become almost part of the herd. It is the point where our primary sense of being is either affirmed or threatened. The man with the drawing of the fortress is actually afraid of being killed. This is a very primitive, deep, feeling. The event that may have triggered the feeling may have been insignificant. A school yard tussle with an older child, possibly, could frighten someone so badly that forever after a fear of violent death haunts him or her.

Jung had still more to say about the psyche. The third diagram he produced is again different. He envisioned the person's entire being, the Psyche, as a large sphere in the center of which the self was buried. The Ego is found at the top of this sphere, looking outward for the most part, dealing with the outside world, surrounded by the buffer zone of the Persona - the mask we bring to our social interactions.

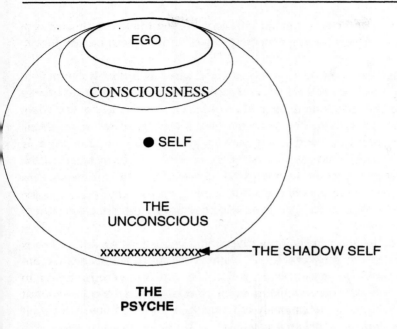

THE
PSYCHE

The self is both the center and the whole sphere, it is the germ of all that one can be - but often the Ego is unaware of this, and so the possible human cannot emerge fully. The initial encounter made by the Ego with the Self casts a shadow. The 'shadow self' is made up of all those parts of one's selfhood that one would prefer not to see in one's self. Yet Jung claims that if we can face that shadow it can become a source of great psychic energy.

Jung also said a lot more than this, and I would willingly go into all the ideas except that it really doesn't have much to do with our task just now. I wanted you to be aware of these ideas because in each case Freud and Jung stress that there is an enormous amount of our lives that is unconscious and that the conscious world seems to push it into the depths -- to repress it, in fact. I also wanted to be able to show you 'pictures' or diagrams of the mind that show how we think it may work. I did this partly because I feel pictures are more memorable, and partly because of our own previous exercises which involved pictures.

Take the time, now, to write about your thoughts about all this information. Does it make any sense to you? Which pieces seem to be useful, and which not? Look at Jung's chart of the four areas of feeling. Where do you fit in? Are you an extrovert or an introvert, do you think? A thinker or a feeling person? One who trusts concrete senses or one who trusts intuition?

This brings me to our next group exercise which is probably familiar to you in some guise or another. It works best when the group sits in a ring with no table or obstruction in the middle of the circle. The leader takes two pencils, passes them to the person to one side, declaring, "They are crossed" or "They are uncrossed," and asking the next person to do the same as he or she passes the pencils along. The leader then corrects those members of the group who declare crossed or uncrossed incorrectly, until sufficient members of the group have understood what is going on. Ideally, one stops the exercise before anyone feels embarrassed, but not before people have expressed puzzlement.

In the exercise the pencils are a diversion. What is being referred to is the condition of the speaker's legs. Nothing is said other than 'they are crossed/uncrossed' yet most people will fiddle with the pencils, trying to work out a code that concerns the innocent objects. Try, after a few rounds have been completed, ostentatiously crossing your legs, and you will be astonished at how many people miss the cue.

What this exercise can show is the extent to which we allow ourselves to be focused on the conscious side of life, and ignore the powerful body language that is usually unconscious. In a group of college students, for example, where young men and young women are doing the exercise, it is astonishing to me how long the exercise can proceed without everyone solving it. I would venture that at college age one of the things that is most frequently on one's mind is sex. Legs, especially in warm weather, are very visible items of physical attractiveness, quite apart from their proximity to the genitals. Yet we are clearly capable of repressing what we see when we are given a puzzle to solve. In our lives we can do the same thing: we focus on details and forget the deep feelings. A man I worked with once told me that in dealing with the emotionally disturbed, one should listen to the words, certainly, but one should also hear the music. What one thinks is going on is not always what actually is happening. An example of this is well known to teachers who sometimes find that the pitch of voice in which a question is delivered can influence the answers students will give. "Is the answer seventeen?" voice pitch rises, "or is it twenty-two?" Voice pitch falls. If a teacher makes a habit -- and the habit is usually unconscious -- of stressing the correct answer in a certain way and the incorrect answer in a different way, children from the first grade on become remarkably adept at learning the tone of voice rather than how to do the math problem. The teacher can't understand why the students do so badly on their homework assignments and yet do so well in class, and often the answer is not far away.

When working with third to fifth graders I became very quickly aware of how they tried to get me to give them the answer to a problem rather than working it out for themselves. It made sense. At age eight any child has a wealth of experience in getting adults to do what he or she wants. It makes sense to use that expertise rather than the less well developed skills of math, reasoning, and so on.

Other versions of this exercise are the numbers game. The leader places cards or objects on a surface and asks, "What number is it?" The group gazes at the objects and tries to make sense of them, yet the real number is indicated by the number of fingers the leader extends from the hand resting next to the objects, Again, the diversion is supplied by objects and the message from the body is ignored.

We are very good at ignoring our bodies.

We are trained to suppress them. No time for lunch, we say, and rush off to the next meeting. The alarm goes off at 7:00 am, it's winter, still dark outside, but we must get up and go to work. And we do. Our poor bodies, which respond to sunlight in order to wake up, just have to cope. Waking up in summer is never a problem for most people, because the body responds to the sun -- which is what wild animals and birds do. But in winter it's a different story. This gets right back to the previous discussion of biorhythms. If we can ignore our bodies, we can certainly ignore our unconscious promptings.

This leads us into the topic of psychosomatic illness. Psyche -- the mind -- and Soma -- the body -- often coexist uneasily. In psychosomatic ailments there may be nothing physically wrong with the patient, but pain is nevertheless experienced. This can rapidly lead to complications which are very harmful. An example might be of the hypochondriac who is always afraid of some deadly disease to the extent that he or she lives on patent medicines, fears to take proper exercise, and in all probability shortens his or her life. The fear of being ill produces a slew of symptoms, many of them imagined. What needs to be looked at is the fear itself, not the symptoms. This not always easy since the hypochondriac is often very emphatic about being ill and will refuse to entertain any other idea. If the exercises show how we suppress our knowledge of the body, the hypochondriac does the opposite - forces mental insecurities into physical expression. The body is forced to show the mental distress of its owner.

Here is another example. Work done by two colleagues, currently in Texas, indicates that when men are in mental anguish in the more macho southern part of the U.S. they are much more likely to complain of physical symptoms than mental distress. A man going through a messy divorce is much more likely to report a damaged shoulder, say, than seek out a counselor. It is thought that the Southern cult of manhood simply will not allow men enough space to admit mental distress. The psychosomatic illness is sometimes known as 'hysterical' illness and there are countless versions of it in circulation. To have butterflies in the stomach is quite natural when one is nervous, but to vomit each morning before going to school may well be a sign of nerves, fear about classes, or apprehension about classmates. In such an instance it makes absolutely no sense to treat the symptom only. An antacid is not going to calm the terror that produced the vomiting.

This extends into everything we do. We do those things that we enjoy far better than those we do not, and those things we do not care for we may find we simply cannot do at all. "I can't dance!" claims the shy man, and immediately he becomes excessively clumsy. Male impotence is also thought in the majority of cases to have more to do with apprehensions about sex than with any physical disability. But the fact is that if the penis does not become erect when expected, the individual then can suffer agonies of self-doubt and shame. That can make the next encounter even more frightening. Often what is needed is mental reassurance. I give this example because sexuality is in all probability one of the few central drives we can identify. If fear can inhibit such a vital function as that, then we overlook psychosomatic disorders only at great risk to ourselves. The fear may have been repressed, but the body presents the symptom back to us, whether we want it or not. We cannot overlook or repress all our fears because they come back to haunt us in these various ways. We can deny that we are troubled, but if our bodies will not keep the secret, then we can only deceive ourselves.

What does this mean? It means that the conscious mind is not all of who we are, and we must be aware of the underlying currents of our being. And this is an important reason for us to continue to work at digging into the unconscious and unearthing what we find.

CHAPTER SEVEN

One of the things Jung suggested was that if we had a map or guide to how our minds work, it might help us deal with the idea of rhythms and changes in our lives. If we know roughly what to expect in our personal development, the whole process becomes much less threatening. Here is a comparison. If I go with my friends and get drunk, I know that I'll feel giddy, act silly, and the world will seem bizarre. The next morning I'll have a headache and that will teach me to go easier next time. The experience is not deeply threatening because I know that my normal state of mind will return. Imagine, though, that you wake up feeling drunk one morning and you have done nothing to bring this about. As the day continues, you remain intoxicated. The next morning you *still* feel drunk. The entire episode becomes much more threatening because you don't know how it happened to you or when it will end. The situation is out of control. Another example would be at the amusement park. Many people love to ride the roller coaster. As one ride ends, you can see children jump out and say, "Let's do it again!" But imagine if the ride did not end, if it went on for days and days?

Jung's idea, it seems to me, was to give us an indication that we will all go through changes and that these changes occur in certain way and at certain times, and then the situation stabilizes. This is like knowing that the roller coaster ride will end. It can be very reassuring. I suspect we need that reassurance very much.

Why do I say that? Simply because in the U.S. it seems to me that we are out of touch with the changes we can expect in life, and that this has a certain amount to do with popular culture's images of living. Looking at a movie or a T.V. screen almost anywhere in the U.S. in the 1990s, we see beautiful young people and happy endings to love stories. Any screenplay writer will tell you not to write anything for Hollywood that doesn't have a happy ending. It simply won't sell. The media, much maligned as they are, seem to feed us a mixed offering that emphasizes youth and happily ever after - usually achieved before the age of 25. The top grossing movie in 1991 was *Pretty Woman*, a shameless variation on the Cinderella story, which has Julia Roberts as a prostitute with a golden heart hitching up with multimillionaire Richard Gere. Happily ever after. Fade out. The problem with such stories is that they are not only very unlikely, but that they assume that after boy meets girl and true love reigns, that life's struggle is basically over. Try telling that to the 35 year old married couples with kids, mortgage payments, impending job layoffs, medical payments, and car payments, who can't get any time alone except for late at night when they're too exhausted to talk. Life does not end with the wedding bells and 'happily ever after' because the years that follow are as demanding as anything in the teenage, post-pubertal years. We have dozens of movies about 'coming of age' and 'first sexual experience' and almost nothing that prepares us for the radical reassessments that we will have to make if, for instance, we produce children.

The perplexing business of seeing a child grow and develop is doubly strange because not only is the child changing fast, but we ourselves begin to think about our own childhoods, or our parents, and what that means. Just as we get used to the child as a creature in a cot, it begins to crawl, then to walk, then to talk, and *then* it begins to challenge our decisions! That's all in about two years. As the child grows we worry about it. Why are you so late coming home from school? We've been worried... Have you done your homework? We become our own parents. As we see the child giving replies and telling us not to worry, we can hardly fail to remember when we were children, annoyed with our parents' continual questioning. We cannot fail to see that this is an area of consideration that popular culture has not bothered to train us for, simply because it has been too willing to sell us love stories.

There are, for example, very few stories that cover menopause in men and women. I can count a handful, aside from the comic figures that are unhelpfully ridiculed in sitcoms. Yet menopause will happen to all of us, unless we die before reaching it. It is also a fact that menopause hits males extremely hard in their self-esteem, leading to a leap in suicide figures in this age group. It seems that when men are made aware that their bodies are aging, and that life from menopause on is going to be less glamorous than the early years, that despair can bite deeply. Menopausal men may discover they do not believe in their work, or even like it; that they are no longer sexually attractive; that their bodies are no longer as sexually reliable as before; that their children need them less and less; that their friends are distant, lost in the scramble to climb the ladder of success. Their spouses may be estranged, too, and child support payments may seem to be the only familial claim on them. I emphasize the male menopause because it is hardly acknowledged in popular culture. Female menopause has a whole array of considerations that it brings with it also, but it has at least some public recognition. I would contend that if men and women were more aware of this time as a time of crisis, then the sense of hopelessness, of no-way-out that must lie behind the high incidence of suicide, substance abuse and such -- can be minimized. If menopause hits at 50, one can expect between 25 and 35 more years beyond that. Many of the world's finest thinkers did not begin to hit full stride until 50, after all, and I include Freud and Jung.

I am suggesting that Hollywood, and the T.V. channels, and our youth-oriented culture, have sold us short, yet again. We accept their version of reality at some risk to ourselves.

Jung suggested a more continual development, which he derived from mythology in which he considered the real wisdom of mankind to be contained. In *Man and His Symbols* he draws upon the myths of the Winnebago Indians, and in particular the work of Paul Radin and his book *Hero Cycles of the Winnebago* (1948). Jung takes the four stages of development outlined by the Winnebago and develops them for men and women. The Winnebago stages look like this:

1. The trickster
2. The Transformer
3. Red Horn - The Hero
4. The Twins

The four stages -- archetypes as Jung called them -- evolved as parenting guides among the Winnebago as well as being a personal preparation for what the young person must expect in coming to maturity. (Ken Edgar has some interesting things to say about this in Arthur Lerner's *Poetry in the Therapeutic Experience*.)

When the child becomes aware of the ability to outwit the parents, he or she is in the Trickster stage. At this point the child will love stories in which a small figure outwits a larger one. "Jack and the Beanstalk", Brer Rabbit stories, and so on, are the tales that will appeal. It is at this stage that April Fool's Day can become nightmarish for parents, and trick or treat a whole new area of concern.

The next stage, that of the Transformer, is probably best characterized by an interest in constructing -- model airplanes, Lego houses, and so on. It is also the time at which story writing and telling becomes of interest.

The hero, Red Horn, is roughly equivalent to Superman, Superwoman, or a sports hero. There is a time in any child's life when he or she will identify with a hero, often an action hero rather than an intellectual hero. The Saturday morning wrestling shows on T.V. seem to have audiences that are filled with enthusiastic children, most of them aged from 10 to 16. The hero identification seems to fit.

The fourth aspect, The Twins, represents the dual values of power and intelligence, and the stage involves the balancing of these twinned characteristics. In the Winnebago myth, the powerful twin succeeds in dominating the intelligent and caring twin, and the subsequent abuse of power caused both to be put to death. This overtly moral statement applies very neatly to the situation of the adolescent who frequently has more power than he or she can use wisely. One has only to think of the numbers of young people who kill themselves with cars, or who run up against the law, to realize this figure has some validity to us.

Jung went on from this idea to build up the four stages of men and women as he saw them. These make fascinating reading, but they are also open to energetic debate. I mention them in case you want to pursue this further. They can be found in *Man and His Symbols*. My point is certainly not that we should embrace Jung's ideas unquestioningly. It is, rather, that we should be aware that we can expect to go through many phases, some of which are going to be less easy than others. The important thing for us to realize is that there *will* be changes. One cannot treat one's grown up child in the same way one responded when he or she was 5. It is neither practical nor healthy. If the child is strong-willed, this will lead to open confrontation, and if the child is weak-willed or depressed, the result will be an adult who behaves like a five year old! Jung's ideas, whether we like them or reject them, certainly seem to take the idea of a spiritual journey very seriously, and that is at least one reason why they are worth considering. We are all on a journey, and nothing remains the same for long. What can be more repulsive than the cliché of the wealthy older man chasing around after teenage girls who in turn use him for his wealth? What could be less appealing than the aging woman, overly made up, dressed in clothes thirty years too young for her, attempting to attract naive young men? Both are examples of those who have refused to admit to the passing of time, and have clung to the stage they feel they need most.

The Winnebago quartet applies in different ways, too. Consider the young man at his first real job, in his first encounter with an authority figure. He may well regress to the level of trickster, and become the office joker. Or as he grows he may discover that he gains great satisfaction from restoring cars or machines. He could be said to have chosen the role of transformer, as an adult, and may spend his life there. Not many of us make it to hero status, but on a Saturday night, after a few beers, it is amazing how many men and women seem to become heroes in their own eyes. Men, typically, will tend to do such things as race their cars down the street in order to prove their heroic status.

As for the twins, I suspect that most of us get there eventually at some point in our lives. We realize we have some power, but we also realize that it has to do with responsibility. Telling the boss exactly what we think of him is certainly possible, but not to be recommended if we wish to remain employed. At different times, we can expect to recapitulate the stages.

How can we be prepared for our own stages of life? That is not easy to answer, since it has not been established yet how many stages we can expect to face, or what they are. One way to prepare ourselves, I think, is to try this next exercise. Write your own obituary. You can be outrageous if you wish, but the exercise will mean more if you can attempt to be realistic. Possibly you have already been through many stages, in which case, write about them. When you have finished, see if you can divide your life up into stages. One young man did a very witty version of this in which he gave his life "phases". His Blue Period (named after Picasso's early artistic experiments) was a time when the young man was unhappy, or blue, and so on.

A quicker way of doing this exercise is to take a large sheet of paper and draw a line of life. The line is like a graph - it goes up for the good times and down for the bad times. Put in dates and a brief explanation of each point on the graph. Then project into the future.

Here is a fairly typical 'line-of-life'.

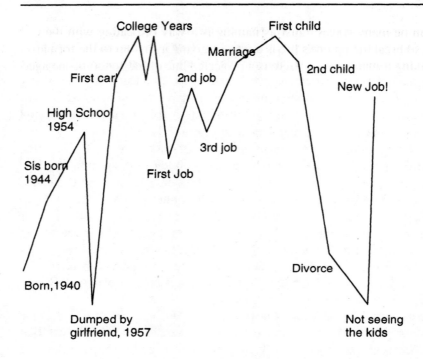

Depending on the nature of the group, this exercise can work several ways. The first and obvious way it works is that it tells all the members of the group what has happened in each person's life and what the hopes for the future may be. For the individual it can be a relief to be able to say to the group exactly what he or she has been through without having to dwell on details. Each of these points is an event, not necessarily a 'phase of life', although one can use it to realize that life is a continued series of ups and downs, not a straight progression. Often it is interesting to note that early events such as "dumped by girlfriend" may actually plummet lower on the chart than such things as divorce. The first shock can often be the greatest. It can help us to see all the events lined up, since this can put a better perspective on where the individual is currently.

The second way this exercise can work for groups and for individuals is that it gives a chance to begin to speculate on when the changes took place, and where the phases of life may be. This is a much more complex task. Ultimately, it has to be said that it does not matter if one comes to a wholly coherent answer or not. What is important is for each individual to see that there can be many stages. Just as naming is a way of dealing with the unknown, so breaking up one's life is a way of giving a rhythm to the formless, thus making it manageable. Here is a projected line of life for someone aged twenty.

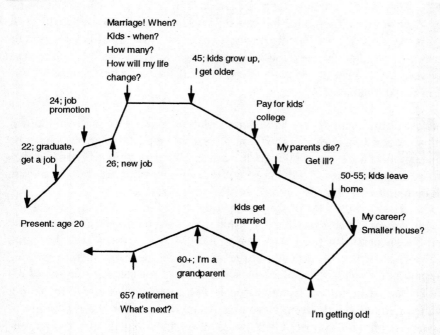

Try to think yourself through the stages. Imagine different stages, such as what happens if the marriage does not work out? Half of all marriages end in divorce. What if there is no marriage? Does that mean being alone? What if your sexual preference is for those of the same sex? What does that mean for one's hopes for children? Many gay couples want children, and this is not a stupid question, since a significant number do get them.

This exercise is never superfluous. I am astonished by the large number of young professionals who reach the age of forty and then decide to have children. Many then find themselves in fertility clinics or adoption agencies, since at that age conception can often be far from straightforward. At the risk of stating the obvious, I will say that many of these people are examples of those who have been so immersed in their other occupations - usually careers - that they have forgotten that life does have certain biologically determined phases. They have bought the myth that they can be young and beautiful almost indefinitely. The truth is something different. Surrogate mothers, black-market adoption - these are partly the offshoots of a failure to see life as a series of chapters we must move through.

Consider what your life might be like at 65. Your job will probably be over - and your children have left home. Will you look back and wish you'd spent more time in the office? Hardly, I suspect. How should this vision of yourself at 65 alter the way you are today? Do you feel you can change the way you are? What about your friends? Will they still be around? What might be your situation?

Most of the exercises we have done look backwards into one's childhood. In this section I have encouraged you to assess the past and project into the future. Like Shakespeare's Jacques, with his "Seven Ages of Man", in becoming aware of your changing body, lifestyle, possibilities, and needs you will be helping to prepare yourself for the struggles ahead.

Variations on the idea of stages are to be found in such things as the 12-step programs. These started with Alcoholics Anonymous and have now been so successfully used that many 'Anonymous' groups use the same twelve steps with very little alteration. And there are many such programs. Al-Anon is for relatives of alcoholics; Al-ateen is for teenage victims of alcoholic families; Parents Anonymous is for parents who admit to having inflicted damage on children; Narcotics Anonymous is for those who are in recovery from narcotic use; Over-eaters Anonymous spells out its own clientele; and so on. I mention this because abusers and abused seem to have one thing in common, they take on roles or behaviors in response to distress, and the comforting thing about these roles is that they give an identity, a direction, to a life that is adrift - however spurious the direction. As one drug abuser said to me, "Life is kind of iffy, you never know how you're going to feel. But with drugs you know pretty much exactly how you're going to feel, and what you have to do to stay that way. Life is real simple!" Obviously, this is a very broad way to look at a very complex series of disorders, but I do feel that it is valid to make the claim that when anyone is afraid of the future, the known evil is preferred. When I was working with disturbed adolescents one of the main problems we faced was that adolescents had frequently been rejected by all those they knew and had ever known. What they had learned was that being rejected and brutalized was the 'normal' state of life. If someone began to accept them the feeling was too new and threatening, so they would frequently do all they could to make sure they were rejected. Then they would know where they were, because that's what they'd always known. One young woman in the first two years of her stay spent a lot of her time kicking walls, furniture and other people. Every home and every adult she'd ever known had rejected her, so she went around thumping everything in sight to see if it would reject her, too. After two years she finally was able to accept that we wanted her there.

This is a variation on a familiar scenario that we've all seen. Girl feels guy is about to dump her, so she dumps him first. That way she is doing the rejecting, and doesn't feel quite so helpless. The young woman who spent so much time hitting and kicking people was actually afraid that once again she'd be rejected, so she went out of her way to signal that if anyone was going to be doing the rejecting it would be she, herself. What lay behind this, however, was a deep desire to be accepted.

If we seem to have wandered from the point, I'll re-establish it by saying that humans crave certainty, and we will do almost anything to achieve it. Twelve step programs seem to work because they offer a series of stages that one can progress through, a support network (a group and an individual 'sponsor' who is a senior member), and a sense of the chaotic void of the future becoming manageable, 'one day at a time'. This last phrase is vital. No one can expect to plot out the whole of his or her life for the future. We can only expect to get through each day with integrity, whilst tentatively allowing for the fact that there will be a future if we deal with today. It is a very carefully-tailored program that will give shape, rhythm and direction to an individual's future. Notice how we are, once again, dealing with aspects of *naming*. Here are the twelve steps:

(1)   Admit helplessness before the drug.
       Admit life is *not* manageable;

(2)   Believe in a "Power greater than oneself" that
       can help;

(3)   Make the decision to turn one's life
       over to god *as one perceives god*;

(4)   Make a searching and fearless moral inventory of
       oneself;

(5)   Admit to god, oneself, and one other the nature
       of one's wrongs;

(6)   Be entirely ready to have god remove these
       defects of character;

(7)   Ask god to remove these shortcomings;

(8)   Make a list of all persons harmed and be willing
       to make amends to them all;

(9)   Make amends whenever possible except where this
       may hurt them;

(10)   Continue the personal inventory and when wrong
       admit it promptly;

(11)   Seek through prayer and meditation to get closer
       to one's personal god, praying for knowledge of
       his/her will and the strength to do it;

(12)   Carry this message to others; *live* it, in all
       aspects of one's life

As you can see this list is a progression that moves from a simple statement of helplessness towards a system of belief in oneself and the universe.
It takes a huge amount of courage to admit to being helpless, possibly because in our culture we tend to idolize those who have control, who are in
power. Admitting to being helpless is for many a bit like admitting complete failure. One man said that before he reached the point at which he
could say it, it felt like he was going to have to admit to being impotent,
castrated. He was a high level executive with an alcohol problem, and so
pride was even more of an issue for him, working in a "man's world" of
business. Making that initial admission can often be a great relief to men
and women in similar situations.

Whatever one's feelings about twelve step programs, with their emphasis on "god as one perceives god" and "the power greater than oneself", they certainly work for millions of people, and continue to do so. I am particularly impressed by the fact that the tasks are divided so that one can see exactly what each task involves. After all, admitting our wrongs (Step 5) is never easy, and takes a major self-assessment. Having done so we are asked (Step 6) to be 'entirely ready' to lose these 'defects of character', and then (Step 7) to "ask god" to get rid of these things. This, it seems to me, is absolutely a correct assessment. How many times have people I know said, "Tomorrow I start the diet" and "Next week I give up smoking". These are trivial examples, but I think that the reason some of my friends are still saying this years later is because they have failed to *name* the task properly. Giving up *anything* means that we have to admit that what we were doing was damaging. That means we have to admit to actively hurting ourselves. Let's spell that out: we have to see that we want to hurt ourselves; or, I have to see that I'm killing myself. If I overeat my life *will* be shortened. If I smoke cigarettes, I will help to kill myself...and so on. We have to admit, in some cases, to suicidal undertones.

The next problem is to want to stop doing it. Many people are quite content to deplore their actions, and not change them. "I know I shouldn't..." they say, and then do it anyhow. The change in attitude that is required is very great. Step 7, "Ask god to remove these shortcomings," is not as helpless as it sounds. God does not magically make it better. What the step conveys is that in order to shed our shortcomings we are going to need a lot of help, and we should not be afraid to ask for help from 'god', our friends, and our loved ones. By breaking a task down to its constituent units, and giving them an order, it becomes much less threatening. As a result, the task can become possible.

As a side note, writing this book progressed the same way. I put off doing it for months, because I insisted in seeing it as a monolithic item THE BOOK, and it felt impossible to proceed. Then I began to break it into named sections, with subheadings. The sections that were difficult to write were those that seemed to have more information than I could easily mold into forms that were compact and easily named. Yet what we are dealing with here is the ebb and flow of energy known as the mind, which is not easy to pin down.

Taking a task, or taking one's life as a series of steps, is certainly not a bad way to do things. Since few of us are exactly where we would like to be either mentally or in terms of our life achievements, it makes sense for us to try to plan the way ahead. Simply hoping that all will magically turn out right is not a realistic option. It is true that some people do win the lottery, but to build that expectation in as a principal component of one's future ... well, that's asking for trouble and disappointment.

The stages of one's life are not fantasy-wish fulfilments. They are a series of turning points that we will have to face. Being ready for what they may involve will certainly help us in dealing with them.

CHAPTER EIGHT

I want to do something a little different in this section. We're going to go straight into an exercise. This is one that is known as 'guided imagery' and in it I ask you to imagine that you are going on a walk, and write down the things you see and do. I don't know who first invented this particular exercise. I encountered it first in England, some years ago, and all I can say is that if it has an inventor, then I hope he or she will forgive the free adaptations I have made of it.

This exercise works best if those doing it feel relaxed, and sometimes, if the meeting is just starting, it is a good idea to let people unburden themselves of the day's frustrations first. A few moments of quiet, possibly a simple relaxation technique, and we can begin. If you have a technique, use it. If not, here is one. Make yourself comfortable, lie down if you can. Close your eyes. Breath in and out slowly, listening to your breathing, then breathe in, hold, and breathe out; pause, breathe in, hold, and breathe out. Keep doing it. In a group setting, I will actually say, "breathe in, hold, and out, pause..." so that the group members are all slowing their breathing in time to my voice. As thoughts come - and they will come - imagine bubbles. Put each thought that arises into its own bubble, and let it float away. Concentrate on your breathing and try to keep the rhythm. Feel your breathing becoming deeper and more measured.

If you are working alone with this book, this exercise may seem difficult. Don't worry. It can be done by tape recording the instructions, then lying down and playing the tape. Read the directions at the same speed as the breathing sequence. And what is all this designed to do? Quite simply, it will help to put you back in tune with one of your own primal rhythms, that of breathing. You will feel your heart beat, also, if you listen for it. Rhythms from within often need to replace those that we find imposed on us.

Often this relaxation exercise works so well that people go to sleep - even those who have, normally, trouble in sleeping. Wake them gently.

Another way of clearing the mind is to do a timed 'freewrite'. Set yourself a segment of time, fifteen minutes is a good amount, and just start writing what ever is in your head. There are only two rules. Don't stop writing, and don't take your pen from the page. If you find yourself with nothing to say, then write, 'I have nothing to say right now...' and keep on until the thoughts surface. You will be astonished how much material comes spilling out. Thoughts you didn't even realize you had lurking in your mind, fantasies, concerns, all are there. Stop promptly when you reach the time limit, and read what you have. You may want to mark sections and ideas that you have noticed as worthy of deeper analysis.

We are now ready for the writing exercise.

Imagine that we are going on a walk. Where would you like to start the walk? You have free choice. Describe the scene around you. What sort of setting are you in? What are you wearing? What time of day is it? What weather? Are you on a path? What's under your feet? You walk on. What do you see? What season is it? Are there any trees or vegetation? In your path you see a key. Describe it. What do you do? After a few moments you walk on. Then you see a bowl or cup on the ground. Describe it. What do you do with it? After a while you come across some water in your way. You can describe that, too. How do you deal with the water obstacle? As you continue on your way the ground begins to slope. Describe that. A little later the ground is level again and you look back in the direction from which you came. What do you see? You continue the journey and after a while you come across a small building. What is it? Do you take a closer look? What do you see? What happens, anything?

This exercise takes a good twenty minutes to write and much longer to share in a group, depending upon the size of the group. Those of you working on your own with this book may wish to use the tape recorder, giving yourself enough time to write the details. If you are working in a group it is a good idea to share all the 'walks' before attempting analysis.

You will certainly be astonished at how varied the walks are, and the varieties of things that are described. Some people will recite actual walks they know and have often taken -- others will be purely imaginary. Some will start off as real places and then slide into fantasy. In all cases there are important details. What one has to determine is the emphasis to place on such details. All have been 'chosen' by the writer, but those which are purely imaginary have been most freely selected, and therefore may be more usefully speculated upon.

First, the time of day, the weather, the season - all these are likely to reflect the present condition of the writer. An evening setting in the fall may well mean that the writer feels that something in his or her life is coming to a close, or that he or she is getting old. The climate of the story will let the listener know whether it is a calm and pleasing situation or one fraught with anxiety. The ground beneath the feet has a similar value. Some people describe themselves wearing heavy boots to tramp over rocky paths, one man described wearing snakeskin boots as he walked down a street in New York City, and a woman was happily walking barefoot on the grass of Vermont. In each case the way the individual felt about the start of the walk reflected internal values, and expectations. The barefoot woman did not anticipate broken glass, and the snakeskin boots did not anticipate meeting mud. The hiking boots, on the other hand, were ready for anything, except dancing. All these aspects have to do with how comfortable the individual feels with life as it is at that moment, and how he or she may deal with it. Footwear can be enormously expressive of one's expectations of the world, as can clothing. Highheels shout out for taxicabs and careful, fashionable, movement, for example. Think of footwear as a basic form of response to the way the individual perceives the world that he or she chooses to inhabit.

As the walk begins, the vegetation can indicate obstructions, usually hinting at the way one feels about people. Hacking through a jungle, for example, could give hints that the person feels stifled by others. A few trees along the path however, would suggest supportive friendships. In this the exercise mirrors the house drawing and its use of trees.

The key can be several things, depending upon the gender of the writer. To both sexes it can suggest the response to an opportunity. Do you pass it by, leaving it on the path, or take it with you? Another interpretation is that it is a symbol of power, since keys open locked places and are therefore associated with those in some authority, and that the phallic suggestiveness of a key fitted into a lock would imply that the key can be a symbol of male sexuality. This post-Freudian symbolic interpretation would be widely acceptable, I believe, to many, if not most, of those currently working in therapeutic settings. This does not mean that the key *is* a direct substitute for a penis. What the key may mean in this exercise depends on the context, but we can certainly surmise that it will tend to reflect the individual's thoughts about male sexuality, and penises, and sex. One young woman imagined her key as a heavy key to the door of a church. It emerged later that she believed that sex should only occur within marriage, and that this was becoming a difficult issue for her as her long-term boyfriend made sexual advances to her that she wanted to respond to but felt she could not. A man related finding a master key that would open all locks. What then had to be discussed was whether this was a wish for sexual potency or a statement of fact. A man with low self-esteem reported a little key for a suitcase. Rusty, dirty, and useless. That was his way of describing this particular key.

Keys are certainly phallic in shape - they are long and tend to have bulbous flat surfaces at the end so we can turn them, making them look like diagrams of erect male genitals. They also are things that we keep in our pockets - close to the genitals - and that radiate power. To get the key to the house used to be a privilege achieved only at 21 years old - the age at which a man or woman becomes legally a responsible adult. When a young person gets the keys to the car it is a major step forward. The car represents freedom, speed, mobility, and yes, sex, or at least the possibility of going out on a date and necking on the front seat... Given the heavy weight of emphasis we place on keys in our society, it isn't unreasonable to look at this key as an indicator as to how we may feel about these things.

The cup or bowl can be similarly interpreted. It has associations to the kitchen, to food, to containers holding food. Since women still tend to spend more time in the kitchen than men, and since women have the ability to breast feed, the roundness of the bowl becomes associated with women in our minds. Whether we see the bowl, then, as a symbol of the vagina or of the breast, may depend upon which way up it appears in the exercise. The way we choose to describe it, and what we do with it, are likely to reflect our attitudes to female sexuality.

I can safely say that I have never had two identical bowls described to me in this exercise. I have heard of cardboard coffee cups lying in the gutter, described by a man who had serious doubts about whether he could trust any woman and who therefore chose to date only women he knew had been promiscuous in the past. There have been Navajo bowls, brass bowls, and from a young woman who was recovering after an abusive relationship, an antique bowl that needed to be cleaned and polished. A woman who had had extensive abdominal surgery, and who had as a result to wear a pouch because her bladder was not able to function, described finding a plain, ordinary teacup, white, dusty, unused. A case could certainly be made for this cup as reflecting a wish for a return to normal health and sexuality. The description of the cup was very unusual because it was so very ordinary.

The water feature of the walk is similarly loaded as to its symbolic possibilities. Water is life-giving. Even the salt water of the sea is full of living things. The fact that we cannot drink that water is less important, on the whole, than the other associations of the sea. Water is almost always in motion, also. Light reflects different colors from the surface, it is always changing. We enjoy water - we swim at beaches and lakes, we take showers as a way of reviving ourselves, and so on. The water obstacle, and how we deal with it, can be seen as indications about how we respond to the realm of emotions, of the body, and also of sex. To give an example, going swimming is hardly an intellectual exercise. That's why it's so much fun. We throw off our clothes and play in the water. The inhibitions remain on land, while in the water we are almost naked, and we see others in the same state. This can be very exciting, of course, and the beach is always a place for young people to meet. Being old, or overweight, is a disaster at the beach! Just similarly, not having a tan is thought of even in our times of diminishing ozone layer as being very unattractive. At the beach one is expected to be a good physical specimen. Water, then, can be said to have specifically sexual overtones.

How we tackle the water in the exercise can say a great deal about how we deal with our emotions, our sexuality, and how we deal with the uncertainties of emotionally charged moments. A woman described encountering a muddy puddle and clambering through trees or low branches to avoid it. At the time of writing, she was in desperate flight from what she perceived as her "messy" emotions and sexual entanglements. A woman going through a divorce described walking past piles of trash, to a black stagnant pool with old oil drums and rusty machinery nearby. When asked about it she defended it by saying she walked her dog there every day. My response was to point out that she chose to go there, and to record it as her 'walk'. Her depression was clear. Merely to respond that the walk was 'real' should never blind us to the fact that we have choices. If she had wished, she could have walked her dog in any number of places. Instead, she chose a joyless and gloomy place since it converged with her inner mood about her sexual and emotional distress. Notice that the water is a dead, stagnant pool. All the joys of life, positive emotions, and sex - all are gone. This was simply a place to take the dog to defecate.

On the positive side, I've had many people report waterfalls and lakes on sunny days, and they have swum, played and had fun. It is in the contrast of such descriptions that individual group members can see themselves a little more clearly. A man who, it turned out later, suffered from impotence, reported meeting a small river that he was unable to cross so he walked along the bank until he found some rocks that he could use as stepping stones. It was not until well after we had finished the exercise that he was able to write about his impotence, and when he did he described first his blank astonishment, then his search to find a way forward, and finally the gradual steps, like rocks in the river, that he had taken. He succeeded in overcoming his problems, too, and developed a satisfying relationship with the woman who had helped him through. A highly intellectual man, he was 25 and entering his first fully sexual relationship. Instead of panicking, he used his intellect to take him through the problem one step at a time. His encounter with the water obstacle was, I thought, an almost perfect mirror of what he was then doing in emotional and sexual terms.

The slope in the walk can be either uphill or downhill. I purposely didn't specify which. Uphill may suggest the thought of struggles ahead, downhill suggests an easy future. The question has to be: how is existence at the moment? How is the future perceived?

Looking back, the next action on the walk, may indicate how one sees the past. A woman described seeing a herd of elephants stampeding past, over the path she had left behind. Another woman remarked that she suddenly noticed little men shooting arrows - all of which she had miraculously and unknowingly avoided.

At this point the time of day and the nature of the path also tend to indicate how the individual feels about the on-going portion of his or her life. The scene at the start of the walk may be idealized somewhat, and thus misleading. By this stage the information may be more topical and closer to reality.

The building that appears towards the end of the walk can mean several things. It can indicate rest, company, possible refreshment, since one could expect it to have those values in the ordinary world. At the symbolic level, however, it can be seen as a tomb, or one's attitude to death. Most people doing this exercise have reported the building as being an old-fashioned hut of some sort, deserted, ruined or temporarily vacant. None have wanted to stay there, although some state that they have been offered food - usually by old people - and then moved on. Possibly the fact that I work with people in their 20s, for the most part, makes my findings biased, but I would expect that people of that age are not really very experienced in death and so are not interested in this cottage of death. The same exercise done with a group of nurses revealed them to be very relaxed around the cottage or hut they described. And that is certainly what one would expect from people who see death frequently in their work. Most people report that the visit to the building is towards the end of the day. A young man provided a walk that ended at his primary school and he played basketball with the caretaker. Speaking about it he regretted the passing of those innocent years, and he supposed the old caretaker who used to be there probably wouldn't remember him. When we applied this back to the young man's life, various connections could be made. He wished for a career as a professional comedian, and was a very playful person in many ways, yet his father was suffering from acute Alzheimer's disease, and this had damaged his young adulthood with the burden of worry. It's not surprising the caretaker didn't remember him, just as his own father didn't, and the young man himself was the 'care taker' who looked after his ailing father. Aged 75 the old man was not expected to live very long, although each day was certainly painful for the family.

I give you this example in detail because the building of death cannot be said, definitively to 'mean' this or that, but rather it exists in each individual's mind in a way that echoes and reflects real issues. It is the bringing forth of these issues, the making conscious of that which was not fully conscious, that is the road to mental health.

Now that we've looked at the guided imagery of the walk, and the similarly guided images of the house drawing, we can take a look at symbols and images generally. The skills that you have now learned in the business of interpreting those images are the same sort of skills needed to decode the images in dreams. Again, I must stress that there can be no direct one-to-one correspondence that says A must mean X. Dreams work in many ways, and the only reliable way to attempt dream analysis is to make one's deductions based on more than one dream. The more the better. For this reason many people keep dream diaries. Odd as it may seem, once one starts re-cording one's dreams, one tends to find that one remembers more dreams than previously. Remember my idea about the rhythms of writing? This is just one example of how the habit can pay off. A note book kept by the bedside is a good way to start, since dreams have a way of escaping from us with each waking claim on us. You might also want to set your alarm ten minutes early so that when you wake your first thought can be of writing down your dreams rather than of rushing to get ready. People who do this report that the recording of dreams has a calming effect that lasts the rest of the day. Personally, I always feel as though someone has given me a pres-ent when I write down my dreams each morning. Even if I have no idea what the dream conveys, it still feels enriching.

There are many different ways that dreams work. Some are responses to outside stimuli. A ringing alarm clock may be translated into a fire bell in the dream, and external noises are fairly easily incorporated into dreams in this way. There are dreams that recap events from the day before, or reflect anxieties about identifiable things that we are already worried about.

Beyond these are the 'pure' dreams which contain few recognizable situations from the everyday world and few people that we know. In these we are in a more rarefied symbolic realm, where things are much less easy to define. Dreams of all these types can be in color or black and white, have music, or not, and allow us to do unusual things.

The next level is the guided dream. In it we can, if we are lucky, direct the course of events. If we don't like the dream, practiced dreamers can cre-ate more satisfying circumstances, enabling them to do unusual things, or even to change the dream. Beyond this is the shared dream. Many well-known cases exist of shared dreams in which two people, independently and often without knowing each other at all well, dream the same dream, pre-cisely. Other instances include dreamers who dream with accuracy about another person's life or day-to-day actions, even though that person may be barely an acquaintance.

When dealing with dream analysis it is as well to make suggestions to oneself and others rather than definitive statements. On many occasions I have found very insightful dream discussion groups generate themselves as a result of the group activities we have been through. Often one dream will spark in someone else a memory of a dream, and so on. Suddenly the group finds itself functioning at a different level from that of ordinary discussion. What is happening is that the members are thinking symbolically, looking behind the images to their potential values. Discussions about recurrent dreams can also be very useful in learning about oneself. Both Jung and Freud thought that dream material came from the most profound levels of the unconscious and that their content was exceptionally valuable, although confusingly encoded. A recurring dream, therefore, is a dream with a message that is asking to be understood, and which is repeated because it has not been understood yet.

If you have had a recurring dream, or dreams with elements that have repeated themselves, take the time now to write about them. When did you first dream this? What did it feel like? Are you still dreaming the same dream? Often? Write about this. Do not try too hard to get meanings just yet. The act of writing the dream will cause you to think about it at a level that is barely conscious, and the value of the experience will come to you in time. Again, writing down the dream is the first step to making that which was unconscious conscious. It's a form of naming. Having named the experience it seems to give the rest of one's brain 'permission' to weigh the value of it.

What do I mean? Let me give a crude example - crude because the mind works in far subtler ways than this. Imagine that you are driving along late one night and you suddenly realize that you have barely enough gas to get to your destination. Immediately you begin to think about what you will do if you run out of gas, you try to recall if you've ever seen a gas station open this late on this road, you start to do higher math based on how far you think your car ought to be able to go after the needle on the gauge reads Empty. You do all this at the same time as you continue driving in your usual fashion, stopping at red lights and avoiding obstacles. Nothing has changed except that you have noticed what the gauge says, although it has been saying empty or nearly empty for some time. A dream is like a glance at the gauge. It engages part of the brain without impairing your usual functions.

The more dreams one has recorded in the dream diary, the more likely it is that identifiable patterns can be picked out, and repeated images can be seen. Since each image or pattern is likely to be in a different context, new light is constantly being shed on the content of the dream. How might this dream material apply to your life? This is the vital question. There are, alas, no easy answers. It is up to you to record, to write, to think, and to write again. The skills you have now, from the guided walk, should help you to be able to 'see' the dreams more easily.

What we have been doing in this chapter also includes something rather important. After our discussions of identity, fear and pain, we have now begun specifically to talk about sex and sexuality. Certainly, it is not really possible to talk of identity for any length of time without mentioning sexuality, as so much of who we are has to do with gender and how we came to terms with the powerful anarchic prompting of sex. Not surprisingly sexuality has been at the center of some of the bitterest disputes in our world today. What homosexuals should or should not be permitted to do is a question guaranteed to raise tempers on all sides. In 1993 the rôle of gays in the military made headlines. Politicians are not usually welcomed by the public if their sexuality is anything except monogamous, married, and heterosexual. One of the things that Islamic fundamental groups have often cited as being an unacceptable part of the Western World is the sexual freedom allowed to women and homosexuals. Alice Walker, the writer and feminist, has spoken out energetically about ritual female genital mutilation done in the name of fundamental Islam, as well as stressing other forms of suppression of women. We would be correct in deducing that gender and sexuality are dangerous topics world-wide, and although less dangerous in the West, are still not entirely open items. Rightly or wrongly, many homosexuals are terrified to admit their sexual preference to any but their trusted friends. And the examples multiply.

The exercise was a carefully-veiled starting point for an investigation of sexuality. At this point, if you are using this book in a group setting, you may not feel safe enough to discuss your sexual impulses. Fine. But you really ought to write about them.

CHAPTER NINE

In the previous sections I talked a little about denial and about the task of naming and shaping one's world. I want now to spend some time looking at the nature of pain.

Pain doesn't have to be vast in order to hurt. It only has to be perceived as vast. It is never a question of how serious the pain is in an objective sense, in stead it is a case of how much of the mind it takes over. A child who is frightened by a dog is, probably, not a major consideration for many of us. If, however, the child feels genuinely in danger of imminent and painful death, then the mental distress is significant. Another example was given to me by the British therapist Peter Wilson, who pointed out that babies often become distressed when they are hungry. To adults this is not really a big issue - we know the child will be fed eventually. To the baby, however, feeding is its whole world, and the absence of food at the correct time is acutely terrifying. "Why else do you think they yell like that?" Peter asked me. It's not the objective size of the pain that matters, but how it is perceived.

Again, a different example altogether may help to show what is at issue. Beating a child may cause dreadful psychic scarring, but ignoring a child - simply not paying any attention at all - can be just as damaging. Sometimes one meets abused children who know that they did not deserve to be punished, and so can come to terms with the situation relatively rapidly. The converse of this is the child who is psychologically misled by adults and who is therefore not sure at all what the mental climate might be.

Whatever the pain is, it has to be unearthed from the repressed memories and dealt with. Sometimes the individual is not even really aware that the pain is there until it has been exhumed. "Why was my father never there?" asked one young man. He had become used to his father's absence and, at 24, had discovered that he had really missed out on something, and he was angry.

When we unearth our pain, we have to realize that part of the healing process is to go through it. "Why should I do this? It only makes me feel worse!" That was the reaction from one young woman I worked with. Like surgery, it's never easy to deal with, but it has to be done. And one feels much better afterwards.

The next pages will discuss various ideas -- using diagrams again -- of how we deal with pain, and therefore, what we can expect in the future when we encounter it. A good starting point is to look at the work of Elisabeth Kübler-Ross. Her highly-acclaimed work *On Death & Dying* (New York, Macmillan, 1969) describes the stages faced by those who have to deal with death -- their own and that of others. She identifies seven stages, of which five make up the central psychological process. They are as follows:

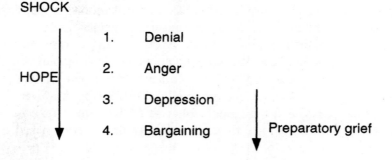

SHOCK

HOPE

1. Denial

2. Anger

3. Depression

4. Bargaining   Preparatory grief

5. Acceptance

Decathexis / separation; Letting go

When one hears that someone close is expected to die the first reaction, after the shock, is likely to be to continue as if nothing has changed or will change. This is denial. When the message finally seeps through that the bad news is not going to go away tomorrow, there is a period of anger that eventually fades into depression as the anger is found to be useless. How thin the line is between "It's not fair!" and "The world's got it in for me!"

As this depression begins to fade a partial acceptance of the situation leads to a position known as bargaining. In this stage the individual hopes and prays for a little more time, a few more weeks then he or she will be able to accept the death. The important point is that the inevitable has been accepted and it is only the timing, not the fact, which is at issue. Finally, there is acceptance in the fullest sense, and this allows the people intimately concerned to let go of the dying loved one, or the dying person to leave the world without regret.

I synopsize these ideas not because we will spend the chapter talking about death, but because I feel it is remarkable how close the stages of dying are to the stages of grieving. Kübler-Ross's work has proved invaluable for medical professionals and patients alike as they struggle to come to terms with death. I contend that the mere fact that one knows that there are identifiable stages, and that the experience will conclude, can be a major consolation. When I sit in the dentist's chair to have a cavity filled, I accept the pain and discomfort because I know it will be over in a few minutes. If I thought he'd be inside my mouth for the rest of my life, I'd certainly not want to sit in the chair to begin with!

The stages of grief may seem simple in the diagram, but I should add that it is always possible for a person to return to a stage, to slip backwards. Anger, in particular, tends to return at different times all through the process.

Losing a loved one to death - facing death oneself - has a great deal in common with how we deal with mental pain carried with us from the past. When an event that is damaging occurs we tend to go into shock and denial. It can be as straightforward as, "I can't believe my girlfriend walked out on me," or as perplexing as, "Why does my mother, who says she loves me, hit me all the time?" In the second instance, if the child is young there is likely to be a profound confusion in which the child accepts the contradiction by formulating the idea that hitting is a way of expressing love, or that the child herself is 'to blame'. This is a way of denying or misperceiving the reality of the situation, and the child is left with a diminished self-image. I want to stay with this example, because if the child is unable to face the fact that what is happening is abuse then he or she cannot progress through the stages. The child is very likely to accept the beatings and claim that it doesn't hurt, that it doesn't matter, that he or she fell down stairs...and so on. Almost every conceivable excuse has been offered by battered children as to why they are bruised, and all excuses deny the real situation. Notice, I am not saying that no child should ever be corporally punished. Sometimes a parent may find a swift smack on the backside to be effective. I am talking here about repeated beatings, viciously delivered. A smack on the bottom may carry a corrective sense; that is up to the parent. Two black eyes and a broken rib are merely the signs of a sadistic desire to damage and humiliate.

The point here is that if anyone, old or young, becomes stuck in denial of the fact, it is very difficult for that person to feel the emotions that are appropriate to the event. Mental pain is caused by an assault, mental or physical, upon the individual. Our natural reaction when attacked is likely to be anger. If I am pushed out of the way while getting on to a bus, I'm likely to feel angry at the person who pushes me. I have choices. I can voice my feelings; I can remain quiet; or I can pretend it didn't happen. If I voice my feelings - and this may not be advisable if the person is likely to be violent or extremely abusive in return - I have at lease registered my complaint. My self-esteem has some consolation. If I remain quiet, but seething inwardly, I am likely to blame myself for the incident. The thought process may go something like this: "Of course, I can't complain, he's bigger than I am. If I weren't such a coward, he'd never have gotten away with it. I suppose I deserve to be pushed around. Everyone does it to me. It's my fault for being a wimp..." This leads to a downward spiral of depression, and lack of self-worth. My third option is to pretend it didn't happen. If this choice is taken, then logically there is nothing to prevent me from reaching the stage where I expect and take it as normal that I am pushed aside. If it didn't happen, how can I deal with it? This choice, and the choice of keeping quiet, require a vast amount of psychic energy. What people who come to therapy discover is that huge amounts of time and energy are taken up in attempting to hide the problem. Once the problem is dealt with, all that psychic energy can be liberated for productive purposes. To return to our example. If I am seething mad at the man who pushed me, I may find it very difficult to think of anything else. I may be unable to read the newspaper, if that is my usual activity on a bus, and I may feel tense and upset. Worst of all, I may feel I cannot show any feelings openly. I will try very hard not to look or act upset. My whole day may be tainted! All that suppressed anger may make me, in turn, rude to my colleagues. The cycle continues in this way.

The healthy reaction - an immediate objection - allows me to pass rapidly to anger, express it, feel gloomy about the manners of my fellow citizens (depression), consider taking a different bus in future (bargaining), and come to terms with the fact that there are rude people in the world (acceptance).

I use the example of myself in the bus line for another reason. If one has to share the bus with the person who pushes one, it is more intimidating to express one's feelings. What happens if that person becomes violent? I'm stuck on the bus with no immediate escape. Strangely enough, that is exactly the situation in many families. Many people report that they simply cannot express their anger to parents or siblings because the other person is right there all the time. Even the bravest of us is likely to find it difficult to speak out, at times, to our families. We may keep our feelings and anger simmering inside for years, often for a lifetime, expending huge amounts of effort in trying not to let it show.

An example springs to mind of a woman, now in her seventies, who had a phone call from her fifty year-old daughter. For nearly an hour, she said, her daughter raged about all sorts of things, events from years before. She just listened. "I guess she had to get it all out," the mother said. Neither mother nor daughter have referred to the episode since, and it has been five years since the call was made. They do, however, have a good relationship. I'd like to draw attention to the fact that the daughter, who had left home twenty five years previously, had finally contacted her sense of anger. She had let it out, and as a result she had been enabled to move on. Unless we feel the feelings, we cannot hope to move through them.

What happens in therapy is that often people arrive seeking help with the weight of their unexpressed feelings. So much inner energy has been required to pretend that all is well that it feels as if life is no longer manageable. Like a person with a huge backpack, at the start the weight is fine, as time goes by and the backpack remains heavy, all other actions become more and more difficult and cumbersome.

The client wants the backpack of pain removed. In order to do that it is first necessary to acknowledge that there is a backpack, and that it belongs to the client. A colleague who worked at The Institute of Family Therapy, in London, frequently found that the most difficult thing in dealing with families was getting the whole family in the same room as a therapist. Each member always wanted to blame some other member of the group as being the 'problem'. This is a version of failing to admit that one has a backpack that needs to be shed.

Once the pain has been admitted by the client it really has to be felt. It is not enough, as one young man did, to state breezily that he was angry with his mother. The anger has to be there. This frequently makes the client very upset and many people leave therapy at this point saying that it has only made them feel worse, so why bother? When the client begins to express real feelings - however unpleasant - progress is being made. A disturbed adolescent girl I worked with repeated to me what had been said to her by one of the other adolescents who had been in treatment for four years. "He turned to me one day after he'd had a really rough morning and said, 'I think I'm having a feeling.' That's when I knew he'd change and get himself sorted out. Before that he was f---ing granite." She knew what she was talking about. When the emotions emerge they are not always pleasant. Anger often is the first step towards renewed self-esteem. It's the feeling that says that the individual deserved better treatment than was received in the past.

Following this discovery there is always a period of reaction in which the client feels responsible for the bad treatment he or she received, and therefore suffers a sense of gloom about the future. This is depression. It's made up of two sides -- the first is the residue of the anger that says that the individual feels hurt. The second is despair that this pattern will continue forever. In one sense no one can feel despair unless that person knows what hope is. Depression is a way of realizing that all is not well, and that it is difficult to decide how to proceed. "Bargaining" is the next step which suggests that there is a way out.

To bargain means that one does not accept the deal initially offered. In the depression stage one felt awful, of course, but one also became aware that there must be something better. Bargaining is the point at which the client begins to see that part of the problem was imposed, and the other part of the problem lies in the reaction that was chosen. So, if we use the example of the abused child again, the child begins to see that the problem came from the parent's anger rather than the child's actions, but that the child was forced to take the line of action of blaming him or herself, and chose to keep doing that. Thinking like that made it easier for the child to accept the parent's unpredictable behavior. There comes a time, however, when this choice of interpretation is no longer entirely useful. The old ways have to change.

Sometimes the bargaining stage can be potentially dangerous. The client who appears after a few sessions and who announces that all is perfectly clear now, and that the sessions should stop is -- and many therapists who have witnessed this will tend to agree -- often seeking to evade the uncovering of deeper pain. A client in this stage should be encouraged to dig deeper since the action of seeking to escape is a form of denial. Under these circumstances progress has certainly been made, but the deep underlying issues have been left untouched. There is nothing else for it but to keep going.

The business of gaining mental health, in my view, should not be to attempt to take the client methodically through the stages with a view of completing all the work in one fell swoop. I like to think of mental discovery as proceeding a little like a spiral staircase. One tends to return to the same problem areas again and again in one's life. But on each occasion one has an extra 360° sweep of experience and perspective as one comes back to a familiar point. One gains understanding as one moves ahead and the problems which once may have threatened to block one's way can now be looked upon from a vantage point of greater distance, and greater safety. Once the therapeutic process has guided the client past the dangers, the rest of that person's life can be undertaken, alone, with renewed confidence. The problems will come round again, but this time the client will know what they are and what to do.

This may seem like a rather sketchy way of looking at the things one may expect to encounter, but I feel that even a vague map is better than no map at all. When I first entered individual therapy my therapist reassured me by giving the following comparison: he said that what we were doing was signing up for a bus ride. He'd been on the ride before, he said, and although my ride wouldn't be exactly the same as the one he'd taken, he knew we'd visit some of the same places -- possibly all of the same places -- and he could act as my guide. This reassured me at the time, all those years ago, just as I wish to reassure you.

CHAPTER TEN

Afer the discussions of stages we have covered, it is essential to add that there is far more to it than my brief synopsis suggests. While Kübler-Ross's stages of grieving and dying are based on precise, observed conditions she met in her clinical work, there are other approaches that need to be considered.

The Jungian schools of thought are different from Kübler-Ross's factual and empirical research in that they stress the idea of archetypes. An archetype has already appeared for us in the Winnebago Indians' 'Stages of Development'. Each of the figures - Trickster, Transformer, Red Horn and Twins - is a Jungian Archetype. Put basically, Jungians tend to believe that all humans tune in to a sort of world spirit, that communicates with us in terms of figures that appear in dreams. These are archetypes. Over the generations this dream wisdom, which can tell us how to deal with life's problems, has been written about, painted, sung about and danced to, and so we have these archetypes in our culture and our mythology. Bruno Bettleheim, in particular in his work *The Uses of Enchantment* has taken folk tales and shown them to be encodings of information that can help the individual in adulthood. He makes extraordinarily persuasive cases for many Old European folk tales as repositories of ancient wisdom that were surely destined to help the village or the tribe with the process of the individual's spiritual growth to full maturity.

This work has been built on by various people. Jean Shinoda Bolen in *Goddesses for Everywoman*, and *Gods for Everyman* has argued that the Greek and Roman stories of the gods are in fact diagrams of human behavior, showing us what we can expect in our family exchanges. Since all the gods are related in the Greco-Roman pantheon, and all of them seem to be constantly bickering over something, the psychological realism of their actions can indeed touch us deeply. Bolen suggests that at different times we tend to choose an archetypal god to be -- that we live a rôle that already can be said to exist in mythology.

John Bly in his very popular *Iron John* follows a very similar path, but he limits himself to one story -- the legend of Iron John or Iron Hans -- and uses it to help explain how men in today's world may have become estranged from their true development. Camilla Estes does the same job for women in her volume *Women Who Run with the Wolves*, taking her information from the folktales that discuss how women reach maturity.

We could add more writers to this list. Linda Schierse Leonard in *The Wounded Woman* and *On the Way to the Wedding* discusses in similar terms how women come to terms with their fathers and with the mystical wedding of properly founded love. In all these works the emphasis is on the fact that our civilization has a highly sophisticated system of tales that could instruct young and old alike, but that the tales have been discarded, lost, or perverted. The blame seems to rest somewhere in the nineteenth century. The Grimm brothers' energetic collection of folk tales was motivated in part by the fear that such tales would soon be lost. Nineteenth century tales had an unpleasant tendency to be overly moralistic in order to teach children to behave. The aim was control, rather than fulfillment. So for example, *Cinderella* becomes a story about how patience and humility is rewarded, as it is relayed to us in its nineteenth century guise. I have already cautioned that anyone who actually chooses to live Cinderella's story is subscribing to a fantasy of how passivity can make one's wildest dreams come true. As a result there is now a "Cinderella Complex" in which women, and some men, buy into the idea that humility will cause everything to turn out beautifully. In Bettleheim's analysis, the tale is quite different.

Bettleheim makes a deeply convincing case that if we look past the surface meaning we can see *Cinderella* as a story which discusses psychosexual development in women. The sitting in the cinders is a metaphor for the time of adolescent introversion that allows the young woman to decide who she actually might be, so that she can move towards meaningful sexual union. Naturally, others may be less than sympathetic with the dreamy narcissism of the teenager. Ask any parent who has had to cope with a girl growing through this stage.

The point I wish to make is that one has a right to be skeptical, but that one also may need to accept that these tales contain a large measure of psychological wisdom. We may find it difficult to accept the idea of the collective unconscious. Yet the story of Oedipus was psychologically resonant long before Freud formulated the idea of an oedipal complex. The essential observation here is that many of these stories and myths do actually dramatize serious issues that surround the process of growing and maturing. We may well ask what relevance such old wisdom has to life in the last part of the twentieth century. I would reply by saying that human institutions have altered but human nature probably hasn't. Since the best images of adulthood our civilization seems able to produce are rather feeble items, we might want to reconsider what we are being asked to accept. Can you name a single, believable figure in popular culture who is mature, wise, and compassionate? There are dozens of rich neurotics -- but is that what we want to be? On the whole we seem to take inordinate pleasure in the conspicuous failure of our rôle models. The newspapers rejoiced when Donald Trump proved himself just another poorly-married business failure. The tabloids revel in the reports that Oprah is overweight. Bruce Willis has a violent temper, and Vanna White, that wholesome and flawless beauty, has had her marital problems. The list goes on and on, from O.J. Simpson to Elizabeth Taylor. Even the previously immune British Royal family has made an unsavory display in recent years.

So who do we look up to? Certainly not real people, it seems.

Does our literature offer any likely figures? Our music, Art?

I have to say that recent Western Art and literature seems to have done two things at the same time. It has emphasized the virtues of morality and maturity while presenting us with figures who feel deeply the crises before them but do not dominate them. The noble failure has become the anti-hero in the process, and values have lain unconfirmed, undefended. Superman, Batman, Rambo, and Captain America do uphold values. Usually, those values are concerned with looking after a helpless but dimly-perceived "community" and protecting something that seems suspiciously like the middle-class tax payer. None of these heroes, however, is wise or compassionate. All they have are prodigious fighting powers. In fact, if we push further, Superman's personal fulfillment is seen as being lamentably lacking. He never does manage to develop a meaningful relationship with Lois Lane, or indeed anyone at all.

The same problem exists for women, as well. A feminist I know commented very bitterly that the women's movement seemed to have completely ignored the fact that for many women, motherhood was a huge part of their identity, containing love and learning in great measure. For her, too many feminists at the fore-front of the movement were not mothers, and seemed only interested in pushing men's boundaries back rather than re-valuing the nurturing and human importance of child rearing. Gloria Steinem's *Revolution From Within* takes on this very point. Ms. Steinem states that she realized all her energies had been directed outward into the political arena, and that her essential selfhood was under-developed. This reminds me of Lenin telling the former USSR how life should be, according to logic, economics, and Marxist thought. The trouble is that the logic did not allow for citizens to be mentally or spiritually fulfilled, merely for them to be fed.

Clearly, we need better guidance than this.

We have confused notions of the stages of human development in our civilization. The Christian confirmation/first communion and the Jewish Bar/Bat Mitzvah seem to be the most visible of the rites of passage. These solemn spiritual occasions are often not as effective as they could be to the psyche of the individual at the center of them, because they are often performed too young. As a result, the rituals lose credibility, or can do so, and the churches and Temples are under-attended. In place of the spiritual milestones that correspond to a real turning point or inner awareness of the individual concerned, we have practical milestones. In this way, we have managed to substitute purely practical achievements for statements of personal initiation. Some milestones that modern youth tend to recognize might include the following: getting one's driver's license, first date, junior prom, senior prom, first time getting drunk, first time having sex, graduating high school, reaching legal age for drinking and so on. These are important events -- times one will probably remember all one's life -- and yet many of them are glossed over as points in life when one finds oneself taking on responsibilities for managing drink, sex, social relations, machinery -- all dangerous things after all.

Recently, my local radio stations have been broadcasting ads about Rolling Rock beer. In a very long ad a man who introduces himself as 'poet, philosopher, beer drinker' praises this particular brew in terms of events that we, the consumers, can be expected to always remember. First date, first car...first Rolling Rock beer. The ad continues, "for some people it's...an important moment...an Epiphany..." I want to direct your attention to the word Epiphany, because what it means is a profound religious experience in which the faithful person is made aware of a closer communion with God and a wider future. That's quite a claim to make for a beer. I take it as a sign of our lack-lustre Christian devotion here in the Northeast that no one has attempted to sue the beer company. Had one compared Rolling Rock to say, a Bar mitzvah (a not entirely dissimilar mystical religious rite of passage) I have no doubt the devout Jewish population of Boston would have declared the ad sacrilegious, and had it removed from the public air time. I may be wrong, however. Does this mean we can look forward to even more offensive ads? Will products be compared to the Crucifixion, or circumcision, or both? ("Good hardware, strong nails and lumber, make even crucifixions less work...") Think about it. How do we value the important turning points of our lives?

A comparison may help here. In a museum in New Hampshire is a seventeenth century Spanish sword. Engraved on the blade in Spanish is a motto that says, "Do not draw me forth without fear: Do not sheath me without honor." The words eloquently attest to the responsibilities of using a deadly weapon, and the possible repercussions. Today when almost anyone can get hold of a handgun, things are different. Pressing a trigger and taking a life is not any guarantee of spiritual maturity, and yet juveniles as young as nine have done precisely that, presumably in the search for respect, wishing to be treated seriously.

In a conversation with me at a workshop, Robert Bly suggested that one reason there is a drug problem in the West might be because an addiction, any addiction, gives purpose to lives that have lost contact with their mythic roots - their sense of living or spiritual progression and personal discovery. I hinted at that in my section on the consolations of rhythm and compulsions. Again, Will Self, the British novelist, speaking in an interview for *Vanity Fair* (August, 1993) mentioned his former drug abuse problems and concluded, "Writing's an addiction, too."

I would suggest that a productive addiction is probably not a bad thing to have in one's life, except that workaholics are seldom either happy or pleasant company. They tend to make poor parents, too. But they do tend to achieve more worldly success than others.

How do we proceed then? R.D. Laing suggested that in order to come to terms with life we have to undergo a schizophrenic crisis so that we can make our way forwards to a balanced world view. The split-mind of schizophrenia, according to Laing, is an essential stage for us all to pass through. Put baldly, we have to come to an understanding of our own unique character and yet be conscious of the fact that the outside world really doesn't care about us and demands that we conform. We have, therefore, to live in two contradictory worlds and yet remain with a sense of integrity. There are 5.5 billion of us in the world. Logically that means that no single one of us can matter much, and we know that. Yet we all have to get up each morning and go to work believing that we do matter. And we do.

This can be a very distressing situation, naturally, and occasionally people will distort the world to fit their fantasies of what it ought to be, and then project their inner fears onto that outer world. Julian Silverman, writing in *American Anthropologist* (Vol. 69 No 1, Feb. 1967) differentiates this paranoid schizophrenia from what he calls the battle with the self. I think that this is a useful distinction, since it conveys to us that schizophrenia can tell us a great deal about mental health, and that in itself a schizoid episode is probably an important learning process we may all go through.

John Weir Perry has suggested something similar in *Annals of the New York Academy of Sciences* (Vol. 96 January 27, 1962). He has identified six types of self which he considers may correspond to the stages of clinical schizophrenia. The stages are as follows:

> The Innocent
> The Orphan
> The Wanderer
> The Warrior
> The Monarch
> The Magician

The healthy psyche progresses through these different rôles, balancing the inner and outer worlds, while the unhealthy mind seeks to adapt the outside world's circumstances so that the individual can indulge in the various dramatic expressions of the inner turmoil.

Personally I like these six rôles, because they ring true. I have watched new employees go through them when dealing with their careers, and I have felt them myself. When I first arrived in the United States I was very much the Innocent. This lasted until I realized I had no contacts and friends to help me, when I became filled with a feeling that really could best be described as The Orphan. In my desire to find out what I could do with the direction of my life, I tried many possibilities. Some were very remote from my life experience and training. I really was a Wanderer at that point. After much wandering I found myself becoming engaged with and committed to certain ideas and causes, which I then chose to champion. The Warrior, in a muted sort of way, was what I became. The next phase, The Monarch, began to arrive when I realized that not all battles could be won, and that there were wiser ways to use power than combatatively. The Magician phase is one that, I think, takes a lot of time to achieve, since one has to acknowledge that there are some things that probably cannot be done, and there are others that one can cause to occur *without* directly doing them oneself. The monarch thinks he is in charge. The Magician knows that he is fortunate enough to have been loaned some power that is bigger than himself and should not be used selfishly.

Often I think what a splendid guide these six rôles would be for anyone working in management, since employees are just people growing up, and they can get stuck at any stage. Some people never make it out of the Innocent stage, expressing pained and surprised bewilderment that management has inflicted something on them. The Orphan may wander about the workplace looking for someone to take care of him or her, and eventually resolve the problem by becoming almost slavishly attached to some figure who is more senior. The Wanderer will have irons in many fires - sometimes too many - and will be looking to see which direction seems to be most profitable. Some people never grow out of this stage as they restlessly join forces first here, then there, hoping to ride upwards by someone else's efforts. The Warrior is the point at which the wanderer makes a stand and declares what he or she is prepared to accept. It's a major step to be prepared to fight for something, and it should not be belittled.

At the same time, some people never get out of this phase, perpetually insisting upon what they want, always in opposition to any change, usually angry at authority. Such a person cannot let go of anger nor make it to the negotiating table, which is where the monarch should be. One cannot negotiate with a warrior, one can only fight. The monarch knows how to win wars without necessarily winning even most of the battles. That is the point at which the Monarch merges into the Magician.

I use these examples because it seems to me that frequently in the workplace one can see conditions that appear deeply schizoid. As a teacher of literature, I can go into a classroom and engage a class in a deeply moving discussion of death, or love, or tragedy. Members of the class may actually make changes their lives as a result of this, and live more rewarding lives. Yet I can walk out of that classroom and be told by an administrator that because of enrollment figures, or budgetary concerns, I cannot teach the class next year. On the one hand I have to believe my work as a teacher matters or I'm likely to give up being an effective teacher. On the other hand, I have to realize that unless I can make my classes wildly popular, however much the students may value them, the administrators will feel differently. Teachers, somewhat naively, tend to believe in education. Administrators, somewhat cynically, tend to believe in money. Which is the real, vital, concern? Many of my colleagues never bother to look closely at this split that they are required to live. The reason, simply, is that between classes, research, and family demands they seldom have time for that "crazy bureaucracy". And that is how it must seem to many teachers. As a result, many teachers have no time to sort out their schizoid employment world, and they remain at the Innocent or Orphan stage, feeling betrayed and alone.

When they go on strike they have entered the Warrior phase. Just as the Warrior risks his or her own life, a strike in any industry can undermine it. During one of the recent teachers' strikes in Boston which caused schools to be closed, many angry parents expressed outrage that supposedly 'caring' teachers could do this to the children. Unknowingly, those parents had identified the precise center of the schizoid dilemma: if one really is devoted to the care of others, then when does one look out for one's own best interests?

Should the teachers win the strike and become somewhat arrogant they could be seen as becoming less-than perfect Monarch figures. Certainly, this has happened in almost every other form of labor at some time or other. The good Monarch, however, is still in a situation of split loyalties. He or she has to be sensitive to those who are ruled, and yet not shrink from swift or even brutal action when necessary. No monarch ever stayed in power by being a nice person, merely. To achieve this balance requires considerable mental fortitude. Oddly enough, Shakespeare can help us, here, if we wish to understand more fully. In his Henry IV plays and in Henry V, he shows us the two sides of Prince Hal's character. The fun-loving and popular prince transforms into an efficient and often pitiless Monarch, who ends up abandoning his barroom friends and even sentencing one of them to death for stealing religious ornaments from a church.

When Henry's army is victorious against overwhelming French odds, one could say he has become the Magician. He does not claim the victory is his personal achievement, or even as a result of his strategizing. Instead, he acknowledges the power of those he has led, who have voluntarily worked with him. If you remember, he allows anyone who wants to leave before the battle a safe-conduct pass. The Magician's achievement is not that he compels people to work for him, but that he encourages others to work with him. Self-motivated, believing in their cause, his supporters can indeed work miracles.

How does any of this effect us?

I would suggest to you that these rôles are not dissimilar from the rôles of the Winnebago Indians that so enthralled Jung. Somewhere between all these ideas the true description of mental growth can be found. All I can say is that it has not been definitively identified as yet. All of these theories, though, can help us if we wish to apply them as ways of naming where a person is, psychologically, and what can be expected.

It is possible that every society needs a different schema of personal development, of course, in which case none of these ideas will be exactly right. That is a risk we have to take. Since our own times have failed to produce anything that is half as helpful as the schemas we have looked at, I think we are justified in using what we have as models for what we need.

Buried pain -- the pain that we have not acknowledged -- proceeds through similar stages as we unearth it. It does not matter if we feel that we are, personally, at the Monarch phase. The buried, ignored pain will push that part of our psyche that is engaged with it right back to the Innocent stage. An example would be the business executive who discovers incest in his family. He does not immediately fall apart and become a childish, clueless, basket case. He may continue to be successful and even flourish, but part of his emotional self will be lost, confused, and very needy. As a colleague said when her father was dying, "It doesn't matter what age you are at when it happens because when it does you still become a little child all over again."

Faced with pain one is likely to show signs of regression. In the writings and dreams of people going through these phases, there are often references to feeling small or being compared to a small object, or needing to be held. Here are some examples that Gilbert Schloss collected in his volume, *Psychopoetry*, which I reproduce by arrangement with Grosset and Dunlap, Inc.

What if, i was thinking, what if i just sat down and started writing something to see what happened....i got out the typewriter and sat down. My face got hot and i started to cry (and it's happening again now) what's so awful and scary about thinking that i might really have something to say, after all and in spite of myself? When you've been hiding all your life (i mean me, of course) it's not easy to start saying HERE I AM, FOLKS, LOOK AT ME. I FEEL AND THINK AND LIKE AND CAN DO THESE THINGS. i'd sometimes much rather say (and the type should be tiny): i'm here and i want you to see me and not go away, but don't look too closely and don't ask me to say anything 'cause i'll get so scared i'll have to run away.

So, Pat, who the Hell are you? What have you got to say? I'd like to say how I like the way my body feels....I'd like to say how autumn fills the lungs of my soul with new aliveness that says HERE I AM, FOLKS. LOOK AT ME.

*　*　*　*

No one ever taught me how to talk
Only how to fluently not say anything
Words come out,
but I don't
I want to own my feelings with my words,
But I don't even know their names sometimes
I have to guess
Someone has to tell me when the words
have left the feelings out
has to show me what my feelings are
And I go back again and try for words.
Second- and third-draft spontaneity is a drag.

*　*　*　*

Patient Conference

-Trial of a child-

"You communicate poorly" they say
    "almost not at all"
"We will help you - this is bad -
    you are wrong"

Frightened-the numbers so large
Faces all staring-
    Are they caring?
    Do they hear?
Do they hear her fear?
Perhaps not at all-

Tell them what they want to hear
Strange language that they can hear...

The pain will remain
As they try to retrain

Give them what THEY want.

                    *   *   *   *

I'm scared
Help me.
Hold me tight.
Use no words,
And tell me-
It's all right
It's all right.

                    *   *   *   *

A Quiet Place to Rest

Bones ache
Mind blown
Gut cast away to the wind
Pathway to eternal security
Roads charred with dirt
Crayoned many colors
Distortions of a formulated personality
World, you're an empty, cruel habitat
Why was I put here?

*   *   *   *

When I am feeling
sour
I will
water
my plants
with
grapefruit
juice.

*   *   *   *

A Worry Poem About Feelings That Are Out of Control

Feelings
        I don't know
     What to do with you
        I am having a
     very hard time
     You overwhelm me
I must find some
        places where you'd
        like to go
Instead of pretending
        You don't exist.

I am so afraid of you
    You are so strong
And passionate
And I am not ready
You are like a volcano
And I feel like a small hut.

Looking at these poems one can apply certain labels to them, if we wish, from the stages we have considered.

"What if..." is a moving description of feeling pain and feeling small. When the writer says "(and the type should be tiny): i'm here..." the lower case 'i' and the emphasis on smallness indicate a stage that is infant-like, defenseless - Innocent, and hurt.

"No one ever taught me..." is surely the saying of the Orphan, bewailing the lack of guidance.

"Patient Conference" with its sense of victimization and desire to get even is close, I feel, to the Trickster phase, and nearly at the Warrior phase.

"I'm scared..." radiates fear and a need to be held like a baby -- which puts it in the Innocent phase, I think, while "A Quiet Place to Rest" with its sense of purposelessness and disconnection is closer to Orphan or Wanderer. The trickery of "When I am feeling/sour..." and its humor, suggest the Trickster who is about to fight back in a more direct way as the Warrior. "A Worry Poem" combines images of smallness "a small hut" and hugeness "a volcano". The emergence of feelings can be terrifying, as we all realize, since it propels us into a new knowledge of ourselves -- in this case the angry Warrior phase. Notice how the fear in this poem can be said to be of the loss of the innocent "small hut" phase. A small hut seems rather cozy to me, very contained. We could say that this is like Anger breaking out of the restrictions of Denial.

Some may say that it is an evasion to use poems by various different people without knowing their backgrounds, since any supposition I may chose to make is likely to be as valid as any other. I chose the poems, however, for exactly that reason. All of them were done by mentally distressed writers, and my purpose is to suggest, merely, that the stages we have discussed may help us to assess writings coming to us 'cold'. It is a possible way of gauging where the person may be in his or her struggles, nothing more.

If you are working in a group with this book, or on your own, now is the time to take a look at your own writings and see if any of these theories and ideas work. Look at the images of size, at the sense of loss, loneliness and abandonment. When do the writings become active or angry? Is this followed by gloom? Remember that the Monarch is likely to be oppressed by what cannot be done as much as exhilarated by what he or she can do. What do you think about all this? Write about it.

You may also want to write about your reactions to the poems. Do they spur any thoughts or feelings in you? Often when I have shown these poems to a group the discussion has taken us a long way from the formal discussion of 'stages', as people have seen themselves in the poems. Which ones seemed most expressive to you? Why? What were the occasions they reminded you of? If you are working alone with this book you will be at a slight advantage since you will be able to spend as much time on this as you need. You will be able to take the time to look through your diaries and papers and seek out similarities.

And then you can write about them.

CHAPTER ELEVEN

A t this point we've probably spent enough time on the stages of development, at least for the moment. We're not finished with them yet, but that does not mean we should beat ourselves to death over them.

The way I'd like to continue is with an exercise. This is one that I first came across in an article written by Mary Clancy and Roger Lauer in Arthur Lerner's *Poetry in The Therapeutic Experience.*[*] I've adapted it in my various uses of it in classes, and now it is quite different from its original version, but I am indebted to Clancy & Lauer's pioneering of the idea.

The activity works well in a group although it can be done equally successfully individually. The equipment needed is as follows:

1. A large roll of paper or big sheets of newsprint paper. Anything big in terms of paper will do, so that everyone can feel free to take as much as he or she wishes.

2. Various brushes, all sizes.

3. Paint. I like to have poster paints, mixing cups, and a box or two of water colors.

The idea is that you select paper, paint and brushes, place the paper on the ground at your feet, and, poised over the paper with a brush full of paint, close your eyes. You should let your mind go blank for a few moments. Then, when the moment feels right, lean down with your eyes closed and make a design. Open your eyes. Look at what is on the paper. Give it a title, the first thing that springs to mind on seeing the pattern. Repeat up to five times. Take a break.

---

[*] M. Clancy & R. Lauer, 'Zen Telegrams: A Warm Up Technique for Poetry Therapy Groups'

Clancy and Lauer call these 'Zen Telegrams' and see them as a way of reducing inhibitions. Whenever I have done this exercise, however, I have found that the activity takes on a life of its own. Often it is difficult to stick to the original assignment and group members start elaborating upon their initial designs, producing detailed, playful and exploratory drawings. Often group members will produce drawings that are exactly labeled with all the feelings that are most intense for them in their daily lives. "Confusion" one woman labeled hers, and the second one which was startlingly similar received the title "conflict". I have found that the exercise takes as long as an hour, frequently, and that much of it takes place in almost total silence as group members look at what they are doing and consider what they are feeling.

If you are working alone with this book, take time to gather the necessary implements and to use them. After your paintings are finished you might want to hang them up somewhere and reflect upon them. Then you should write about them, the way you felt as you did them, and anything they brought out.

On occasions, working with groups, I also have quite shamelessly arranged the exercise so that it can reveal other things as well.

For example, I do not clear the room. I leave it to the group members to make whatever space they need, by moving chairs. Sometimes this means that individuals work bunched together, or one is isolated in a corner. People end up stepping around each other, aware that what they paint can be seen by all, or at least some. People often pair up or form small groups, while others go off alone. I also arrange it so that there are not enough brushes of each kind to allow everyone to have one of every available size. Similarly, there are not enough mixing dishes. I do this not to inhibit the shy members but for another reason. By this stage the group members are well enough acquainted that shyness is less an issue than the fact that I gently prod them towards making their choices of brush, color and place *felt* as choices. Even the simplest negotiation expresses the choices, and since the whole purpose of my approach to therapy is to help people become conscious of their choices, this seems to be a valid way of going about things. The sense of seriousness of the exercise is carried through from beginning to end. At this point the group members know that this is not frivolous but an exploratory process.

If you are doing this exercise alone, or with others, ask yourself how assertive you were able to be in getting the creative space and tools you needed. This will be a reflection of how much you let yourself show your creativity in the rest of your daily life. One young woman kept asking me, as the group facilitator, if it was 'allright' if she did this, or that, or whatever. What I was able to reflect back to her was that she has a habit of asking permission in her life, and that this extended to everything she did. As a result her creativity was less than spontaneous. When we looked deeper she was able to make the connection to her upbringing, in which a strong single mother had kept her in check until the mother had married a man of whom the young woman was a little afraid. Consequently the young woman had felt she had to check everything she did with authority figures, and when the painting project appeared, her old habits surfaced and she turned me into the authority who had to be consulted, despite the fact that I had given everyone in the group almost total freedom. In the end she was able to complete the painting by linking with another group member and working together, checking from time to time with her painting partner. I use this example to encourage you to look not only at the painting, but also at how it was done. How much initiative did you allow yourself? Write about this, too.

It could be argued that this exercise makes the process involved seem very conscious. The result would then seem to have more to do with the ego showing itself off instead of the unconscious emerging. I would agree that the ego is involved -- but then the ego is always involved at some level unless the individual regresses to preverbal infant level. At such a level a painting, or even the ability to follow instruction, is not to be expected. What tends to happen in this exercise is that group members are able to project their feelings onto the picture they produce and then explain the feelings. One young man started with a line that he entitled, with great literalness "squiggle", and then as he produced more pictures he became more oblique and more elusive. The papers filled with whorls and lines which gradually became more and more charged with sexual imagery, which we identified in discussion later. The paintings were still enormously abstract, but the sexual content was undeniable. He wrote later: "It was such a relief to paint those pictures! You are right about the sexual content. My sex life has been rocky; I want to have sex, and my girlfriend wants it, too, but I can't do IT..."

A young woman started with very abstract designs and became slowly more concrete in her pictures, the last of which was a picture of a church with a statue of the Virgin Mary on the roof. Not a deeply religious woman, we talked and were able to make some connections. Later she wrote about her fear of sex before marriage. She had in fact been conceived before her parents were married, and her father had later abandoned the family. Later, her mother had left their home in order to be with her new lover, leaving the young woman resentful and having to care for her younger brother. Herself a practical 'virgin mother' to her brother, the homelife she craved in the church, the house of God, seemed reflected in this most 'conscious' of paintings. As this emerged she was able to write about her desire for excitement in life, and yet her fear of the unknown, and her ambivalence about her chosen career as a primary school teacher. Her early life had been spent caring for others, and now her adult life seemed to be following the same course. Yet she wanted excitement!

Here there seemed to be a clear example of the childhood fears and experiences being carried into the adult's life. The only way to break the chain was to acknowledge its hold on her. The conventional picture had, in fact, been very revealing.

I will continue to discuss this young woman because what was remarkable about the exercise was that, as it seemed to be reaching its end (no word had been said to that effect, but the sense was that we had all painted enough) she quietly began to pick up brushes and containers and to take them away. She washed them, and returned for more. The effect was that everyone else started to dither a little and attempt to clean up. Nothing could match this woman, though, as she slipped out and returned with a damp cloth to clean the floor. In this exercise she had elected herself as caretaker, which is her chosen rôle in her family and her career. No one had asked her to do this, it wasn't even necessary. When this was pointed out to her she was both surprised and confused, since she hadn't realized the role she had slipped into.

In an exercise of this sort, at this point, it is the totality of what each person does in the room that is important. Part of the reason the young woman tidied up was actually defensive. If she did this chore for everyone, then surely we'd like her and thank her. In her thinking this would prevent anyone from asking her to look into her paintings, and see what was there. The unconscious was using some impressive defenses. She did not realize she did not want to have to acknowledge consciously what she already had begun to suspect (her ambivalence about her future career) so her involuntary defenses kicked in.

Often this can be difficult territory for both group members and the group facilitator. On several occasions members have spoken to me about this exercise in ways that were charged with sexuality. In each case the sexuality was not a response to the reality of the situation, but rather a desperate attempt to seduce me into silence, into not pressing the questions that needed to be asked. Obviously, a sexual relationship is neither helpful nor healthful since it is in these instances merely a version of manipulative power play. One needs to be very delicate, and very firm, in such matters, and keep the task in mind. Another vaguely sexual advance that was made to me was an invitation to have dinner and talk about the exercise. It may have seemed innocent, but one of the woman's major issues that she had to face was her weight problem and what that meant for her self-image and sexual attractiveness. By inviting me to dinner she could feel attractive, indulge in her eating, and yet not have to really face her sexuality or her eating disorder. None of this was strictly conscious. I give these examples in order to suggest how incredibly resourceful our unconscious defenses can be in protecting our sources of pain.

This is where we become involved in what is known as Group Dynamics. Before I get involved in this, which should certainly be of interest to those of you working alone as well as those of you who are working with others, I want to direct a few comments to those of you who are working without any observers. You should probably begin to think about your paintings in certain ways, which is why I give the examples from the group experience. Let's start with basics. How did it feel to do the first one? How many did you do? Did you give yourself enough space? How much space did you use? I have seen films of Chinese masters of this art who have used pieces of paper twelve feet wide and twenty long, as they gripped a brush that needed two hands to hold it. If you found yourself moving off the paper and putting marks on the carpet, you could be expressing a need for a wider, larger life in which to express yourself. Did your picture seem different after you had written the title? Were your brush strokes sweeping (which would tend to indicate an uninhibited nature) or short lines (which might indicate constraint or anger)? Did you feel as if you were back in grade school? Did that feel good, or slightly embarrassing? Why? Write about it. Working alone, you will tend to recapture those feelings you had when you used to paint a little less than expertly. This may take you back to third grade, or it may take you back to a class you had in college. What was the circumstance, and how did it feel? Since the exercise starts with the painter having his or her eyes closed, there can be no shame about the technical expertise of what is produced. If you are on your own this may be a positive relief - no one is going to look at your work if you do not want them to. Did you feel you had to 'tidy up' the pictures after you had first produced them? Did you begin to paint more on any of them? Why? Did you add color? When the paintings dry, hang them somewhere and look at them. Write about your thoughts.

One of the things about this exercise that always strikes me is that whether one works alone or in a group there is almost always an atmosphere of seriousness and thoughtfulness as the painting takes place. The people who take their shoes off and dabble on the paper with their feet, for instance, are in a minority. What one does in this exercise is to contact a feeling, often a vague feeling, and then one causes it to be made visible as a squiggle. Once it exists physically, the painter tends to project his or her feeling onto it simply by contemplating the result. Often at this stage the picture will be elaborated, as the exploration proceeds. This enables us to capture and explore very fleeting ideas. The point is that by this stage in our work together you will be in some sort of rhythm with these exercises, and your unconscious will probably be ready, primed, as it were, to deliver your repressed thoughts for your conscious exploration. What may *seem* like mere froth seldom is when once it is examined.

To return to the group setting, the experience as I have arranged it will be slightly different, since it will have an extra, complicating, aspect. It will depend, at this stage, on some aspects of group dynamics. What this means is that what tends to happen in any group is that people will reconstitute psychological situations that have worked for them in the past, for whatever reasons. Thus, every group is likely to produce certain figure rôles, almost independently of what those people are like elsewhere. One rôle is the caretaker. We have already seen that one emerge. Another is the Jester. Someone will *always* make the jokes, I've found, just as someone will always be angry and express it. Sometimes the two rôles merge in the same person. Someone will always be the fragile soul, and someone else the conformist, who backs up everything the leader of the group says. These are not rôles in the same way that the stages of development we have already covered can be seen as rôles. These are more localized, usually, although the two different aspects can merge.

Group dynamics can be explained as follows. Frequently, I have observed families or groups in which all seems normal apart from one member. This member 'acts out', that is to say displays publicly, the upset in the group. If we return to the young woman caretaker, we could say that what was wrong in the family was that the mother was not being a mother and looking after the children. The child, then, had to 'become mother' to her own rather helpless and confused parent. The child took on the rôle that was available, needed. Similarly, boys become 'man of the house' in the absence of a father figure, and are capable of acting with surprising maturity if called upon to do so, and display formidable jealousy if the mother becomes sexually interested in a man.

In a remarkable example of this dynamic, a woman in one of the groups was able to admit sexual abuse experienced as a child at the hands of an uncle. The men in the group were outraged. One, who had done time in a high security prison, volunteered to 'fix' the perpetrator, so he 'wouldn't walk again'. He was quite capable of doing the deed, and clearly it was necessary to calm the situation. What had happened was that the woman had managed to make the men express her own anger at her uncle. As a result, she didn't have to feel that anger, let alone think of how she should act in the future. She had literally handed her problem and her emotions to those who could express them better. Logically, it made no sense for the man to cripple someone he had never met -- risking another substantial jail sentence -- for a woman he didn't even like very much. He had given her the nickname 'Princess' because he saw her as fastidious and distant -- yet when the Princess wanted something he responded as if she really was royalty. The power of the group dynamic was such that he would literally have risked years of his life for her. The situation told me more about his self-image and needs than about her feelings. It also demonstrated how emotions can be pushed onto those to whom they do not rightly belong.

A simpler example is that of the bully. The bully nearly always is sadistic because he or she has been treated cruelly. Rather than change the pattern, the poor helpless bully goes and picks on a more helpless victim, human or animal. Why? The reason is that there is relief from pain in being able to look at another and say, "at least I feel better than him!" This crude scapegoating is as old as sentient life, I suspect. Even antelope shun the sick and helpless of the herd, leaving them as the natural victims for predators, making them the sacrifices as the rest of the herd proceeds in relative safety. The sacrifice means that the rest of the herd can relax a little, and the fear diminishes temporarily. Ultimately, they all must end up, at some point, under the predators' teeth, but for the moment, they know it is not their turn, but the victim's.

To return to the exercise for a moment, who in the group took the position of 'outsider'? Who moved off to a private corner to paint? Did anyone? Was there a joker? What was going on in the room? And why do you think it happened that way? If you are not in a group, think of your office or workplace. Who are the secretive, alone figures? Who are the gossips and who do they victimize? Is it always the same person? Who is the angry person in the workplace? Remember, anger can be overt and confrontative, or it can be indirect. Who is the office clown? In some offices I have noticed that the scapegoat is often the copy machine: it is kicked, abused, sworn at, dismantled by people who normally can barely change a light bulb who swear they'll 'fix it' this time, and it is blamed for everything from A to Z. "I would have had it done if it wasn't for that ------- copy machine!" This is an excuse that really carries no conviction at all, to anyone.

Within therapeutic groups, the situation is a little like this, also. I have been in groups in which one member has been consciously the 'outsider'. One such person was also socially a little clumsy and had a harsh, grating voice, so that much of what he said was not only poorly timed (he interrupted others) and a little removed from the topic at hand, but it also sounded insensitive. He quickly found himself the outsider despite all efforts to bring him into harmony with the rest of the group. Although this was disappointing in many ways, he actually grew to love it, since he was receiving attention, albeit negative attention. A profoundly lonely and lost individual, he had arranged it so that he received some form of recognition, after all. The effect on the rest of the group was that it gave them all the impression that because this one man did not, in their eyes, 'get it', then they themselves must be better, brighter and more sensitive. As a result of this the other members did absolutely outstanding work, together and individually. Without conscious acknowledgment everyone was able to receive at least part of what each individually needed. The lonely outsider became convinced that he was more relaxed than the others, and so felt better about himself, and the rest of the group was spurred towards excellence.

I do not want to spend a huge amount of time on the vast topic of group dynamics. I want, here, merely to point out that people in groups are not the same as people individually. We tend to externalize our inner conflicts and put them onto others. If we can decode this we can make considerable progress. I'll give an example. An acquaintance of mine some years back was very keen on dining out. He and I would meet in restaurants and sample the specialties of the place. I began to notice, however, that this man was usually rather antagonistic towards waiters. The longer I knew him, the more pronounced this became, and I eventually gave up going to restaurants with him because there was bound to be an argument. At cafeterias, at private dinners, at take-out places there was no problem. I pondered this until one day I was in a restaurant with two emotionally disturbed adolescents who were under my care. Early in the meal they began muttering about the waiter, and before we had reached the entree there was barely-suppressed hostility, grim looks, and muttered threats about what the two young men imagined to be slights by the waiter. This gave me a clue to their psyches, and to my acquaintance's. The level of anxiety that seemed to be produced between the placing of the food order and its arrival was directed at the waiter. Not at the cook, who after all had much more control over what appeared on the plate, nor at the owner whose finances might dictate the size of the portion -- but at the waiter. It was a classic case of blaming the messenger.

As I worked with the two adolescents I began to realize that they had both been emotionally and physically deprived, and that food, who provided it, and whether it could be trusted to be good, were major areas of uncertainty for them. Their anxiety must surely have been produced many years before as a consequence of repeated poor parenting at a very basic level. Food is one of the most basic requirements, certainly. The anxiety, which properly belonged as an emotion expressed towards a parent-figure, had never been expressed. It is difficult to tell our parent or parent-substitute that one does not trust him or her, especially when one is small, defenseless, and hungry. The emotion is forced to go wherever it can -- and the waiter was the unlucky recipient.

My acquaintance had, it turned out, a very similar problem. As an infant he had lived half the year in England and half the year in Italy, and his mother, who was Italian, cooked Italian and English recipes at her home, while in Italy the family cook produced the meals. Very young my friend had announced that he would only eat certain things - bread, mostly - and had stuck to that. His resentment at seeing others eat what he did not trust, complicated by his feeling towards a mother who seemed to epitomize the constant changes in his life, had marked his emotional responses to food very deeply. Himself, he did not see the problem. It was in the feelings he projected onto the waiter that the clue could be seen.

This is very close to that old truism that: "what we hate in others is the thing we hate in ourselves."

Again, the person who has trouble with the boss, or with authority figures generally is almost certain to be projecting onto others an unreconciled conflict with a parent-figure. This is not to say that arguing with authority figures is bad. Far from it. In the seminar room I note with delight those who challenge what I say. Often this means that the relationship with the parents has been sufficiently open, honest and safe that the child has no qualms at all about saying what he or she believes. Sometimes it means that the parents have been so obviously inept that the child has learned not to be automatically deferential to elders unless they prove themselves to be more knowledgeable. The people who give the most trouble in the classroom and the workplace are those whose doubts about their parents were never expressed or explored, and consequently any available substitute will do. Sometimes I think of human beings as a little like loaded weapons. If the correct target is unavailable, or too risky, a substitute has to be found, and blasted.

This is certainly held by some to be an aspect of that most brutal of crimes, rape. Rape is about sex, certainly, but it seems that it is also much more about violence and the humiliation of the victim. Since many rapists do not ever get a close look at their victims until they assault them, and since rape seems to have no upper or lower age limits, it can be argued that only a very few cases have anything at all to do with the appearance or 'provocative behavior' of the victims. One is left with the loaded weapon of emotions as a theory -- that the rage or anger against a certain woman (or man) is being acted out upon others, years after the events that caused the rage. Eldridge Cleaver's chilling confessions in *Soul on Ice* give terrible testimony to the fact that for him, at least, rape was about being angry and black.

The trouble with this displaced rage, quite apart from the physical and the mental pain it inflicts on the innocent, is that it does not deal with the causes that move the criminal, and so cannot be stopped easily. Imprisonment without corrective treatment (and there is precious little in some prisons) is merely a way of limiting the person physically -- until the chance arises again. Many of us are not dangerous enough to be imprisoned, of course, and so we repeat destructive patterns and often it takes us years to understand why.

Now that you are aware of the existence of group dynamics you may want to see if you can identify them elsewhere in your life and work. Which people seem to take on different rôles at different times? Have you ever felt yourself doing this? I'm certain that if we all look at ourselves carefully we'll discover we do it more than we realize. It's useful material to consider, and well worth writing about. Who are the people you know who always seem to need to be rescued, or who are helpless and asking for us to make their decisions for them? What sort of rôle is that? Who are the people who 'rescue' such people? Possibly you do? What would be the reason for that? It's worth exploring in writing.

CHAPTER TWELVE

I want to introduce some other ideas here. We have looked at theories of Jungian stages of development - very briefly - but I have to admit that I consider that to produce an entire volume talking about these stages may not be very valuable. Many people have done just that, of course, and made a fortune in the process. I would advise you, if you are interested -- and you really should be -- to read works by those authors I have mentioned. I'm not sure that a more detailed paraphrase of them by me is needed.

My purpose is not to argue the broadly Jungian approach in preference to any other. Personally, I believe it has a large amount to offer, but it is not the only approach to the way the psyche develops, and my task here is to make you aware of the possible ways that one can see the problems one faces.

An entirely different theory of early development is one that comes from Erik Erikson. He is more empirically inclined than Jung, and follows Freud in the emphasis he places on childhood sexuality. He has developed in his work *Childhood and Society* (Paladin, St. Albans, 1977) a fascinating chart for the development of the child. The chart is on page 77 of Erikson's book. Here it is.

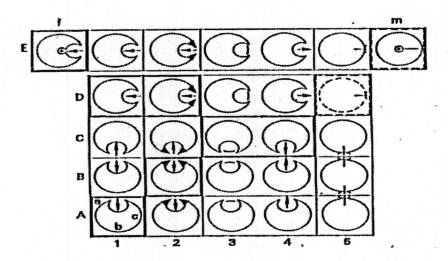

I am going to spend some time discussing Erikson's ideas because I feel they are important. If our task with this book is to attempt to understand ourselves better, then it will be necessary to take some account of how, possibly, we might have developed. If we can understand what the forces at work on us were when we were children, it becomes a little easier to deduce how we came to be where we are now, and how our personal foibles came to be.

Erikson's chart may seem formidable, and it is necessary to focus upon one element at a time for it to become clear. The chart starts at A1. The circle with marks a, b and c is to indicate the child and the three main areas of sensory information: (a) is the 'oral sensory' area, that is to say the mouth, face, stomach; (b) represents the anal and excretory organs, including urethra and the muscles that control both; (c) is the genitalia.

The numbered columns represent an 'organ mode' - how a part of the body can be used, and they are as follows:

1. Incorporative 1
2. Incorporative 2
3. Retentive
4. Eliminative
5. Intrusive

This may all seem very technical, so let's put it all in plainer terms. When a child is first born we have no way of knowing what it is thinking, but we observe that the main activity is centered on the mouth, which is what is shown at A1. Erikson calls this the oral-respiratory-sensory stage, and argues that just as the mouth is eager for food, so the whole skin surface of the child is eager to be stimulated by warmth and comfort. The child lives to be cuddled and fed, and it learns to receive food and comfort. A baby cries when it is hungry or needs its diaper changed, usually, and what the child learns is that mother or parent will feed and look after it. The main mode of behavior is an incorporative one in the first stages, when the child seems to live to feed. If this is disrupted for some reason the child may learn something very different. If, for example, the child cannot digest easily the entire business of eating becomes highly distressing. The child is hungry and yet upon feeding it feels unwell, or vomits, and is hungrier than before. Since feeding is such a huge part of the baby's world, this can be very frightening. When babies cry they do not weep gently, they yell. That should give some idea of the amount of fear they are experiencing.

Again, if the child is neglected and has to wait for a long time to be fed, that experience will imprint itself on the psyche as a "rule of the world" that is carried into adulthood. Erikson maintains that unreliable feeding can upset the child's first negotiation with the outside world, while successful feeding -- which requires love and cooperation between mother/parent and child -- produces a basic optimistic feeling in the baby. This marks the point at which the child learns *trust or distrust*.

Erikson points out that the habitual withdrawal of the nipple, when the mother fears being nipped by the infant's emerging teeth, could be the basis of later disturbances in interpersonal relations. "One hopes to get, the source is withdrawn, whereupon one tries reflexively to hold on and to take; but the more one holds on, the more determinedly does the source remove itself."(Erikson, p.65) It seems to me that this is exactly what I see many people do in their love relationships, obsessively pursuing someone who is busy retreating from them. We learn our patterns of behavior very early in life, and unless we can be aware of possible causes for such non-rational and obsessive behavior, we may be doomed to repeat it, endlessly. Our earliest experiences help to shape our mature actions. We have a duty, therefore, to ourselves to try and look at this distant part of our lives.

From this point the child develops to level B, column 2. Some teeth have emerged, and so the child can bite the nipple. Obviously, the mother does not care for this, and this is usually the time weaning takes place (if not before). There is the pleasure of a new sensation, biting, but also the pain of teething. There is a fairly heavy series of new demands on the child who until now had a relatively simple and straightforward bond with the mother. The child is also learning how to grasp with the hands, and can see better - tracking figures as they move across a room, for instance. Erikson sees this as the stage at which we learn to grasp and hold objects just as later we will grasp ideas and knowledge. Success or failure in the achievement of this stage lays the foundations for the child to feel confident in being able to get what it wants. The act of weaning and the break of the bond with the mother "leaves a residue of a primary sense of evil and doom and of a universal nostalgia for a lost paradise." (Erikson, p.67)

As the child grows it becomes aware of its muscles and of the desire to use them. The child learns to walk and do more complicated actions, and the digestive tract begins to produce a more solid stool. The muscular pleasure of controlling the bowel and bladder and 'letting go' develop within the child a sense of voluntary release and ability to throw away. The child at this point is alternately throwing toys out of the crib and holding on to them tightly in an enaction of the bodily process of satisfactory elimination. This we see in Level C, columns 3 and 4.

This is the stage at which toilet training is introduced, usually. Too rigid enforcing of the regimen can lead to the mechanical orderliness of the compulsive in later life. The person who is so orderly, punctual and precise that the emotional life is unable to develop fully would be an example of this. It is widely rumored that the Swiss, who toilet train infants earlier than most European countries, have the highest adult constipation rate in the world -- seen by some as a toilet rebellion later in life. Certainly the British psychologist D.W. Winnicott saw adolescent bed-wetting as a sign of passive rebellion against a dominant parent. This fits neatly with Erikson who sees this stage as the one at which the child gains some control over his or her body and begins to assert some sense of control. Successful achievement of this stage allows the child to develop a sense of *autonomy* rather than *doubt and shame*.

The development can go wrong, of course. That's why other boxes exist in the chart. The child who had learned that oral incorporation (A1) is a reliable form of love and mourns that loss may seek to incorporate through the anus. Erikson reports not infrequent cases of children who insert objects in the anus or urethra, and so could be seen as regressing to stage C2. He also gives an example of a child so terrified of losing his mother that he 'held on to her' by refusing to defecate, which would correspond to box C3. Holding onto the feces was the only control the child felt he had in his world and so that is where he chose to do his holding on. The obsessively neat neurotic, one could say, is using the control of the anal eliminative process, learned at this early age, as a way of attempting to bring order to a disorderly world.

Levels D and E are concerned with the growing attributes of locomotion and the developing sense of the genitals. Erikson suggests that mobility makes boys intrusive in fact - they like to explore the outside world - and in their genitals. They tend to climb, to push, to pry in a fashion that suggests future genital desires to penetrate. Girls, on the contrary, are seen as regressing to a 'dependent' rôle (at least in our society) of waiting to be penetrated (D and D2) in the same way the child waited for food (A1 and A2) until, much later (at Ef) the goal of genital behavior is seen as pregnancy. Boys also will develop to the same idea (Em) but their behavior will be intrusive, while the girls will tend to take up an 'incorporative' mode, since that is what our society still fosters in its treatment of women.

Notice that Erikson does not attempt to lay down universals of growth and behavior, but only to chart what stages of growth our society tends to reinforce and reward. The active, intrusive female is today more evident than before, but is still hardly a popularly accepted figure in our culture. Similarly, sadists and masochists who could be seen as fixated at level C2 are not made welcome in our culture, although there have certainly been highly sadistic rulers and regimes in our century. Certain types of regression seem to pass almost unnoticed. Compulsive gum chewing, which looks like regression to level B2, is widely accepted as normal, if a touch uncouth in some circles, while the ingestion of milk products such as ice cream, shakes and so on can be seen as a regression to level A1. A colleague who ran a residential therapeutic community used to assert that he could judge the level of distress in the establishment by the amount of milk that was being consumed. In times of distress one tends to resort to early, successful modes of behavior, in this case, breast feeding substitutes. Recently popular jargon developed the phrase 'comfort food' to refer to anything soft, bland, and requiring no cutting or chewing - exactly the sort of food people seem to crave when feeling distressed, and which seems very close to a description of most processed baby foods.

The huge success of fizzy sodas may have a great deal to do with the fact that the carbonated water in the mouth is very exciting to the senses, the gases fill the stomach and give a sense of being fed, and the sugar or caffeine give a mild sense of euphoria -- in fact the entire procedure seems to have more in common with breast feeding experiences than with the flavor of the product. Imagine yourself in the baby's skin. Drinking mother's milk is incredibly exciting, since it is probably the single most sensuous pleasure the baby receives, and gives a sense of instant well-being. Now compare that to the lip smacking commercials of young people gulping down soda. Plain water will quench the thirst more rapidly, and is arguably better for the body, but it never seems quite as vital, somehow. I suspect that the soda manufacturers know exactly what they have hit upon.

Erikson's theories are worth this detailed rehearsal because he emphasizes the early childhood experiences as things that vitally shape the way we perceive the world and, therefore, how we interact with it. This certainly is in tune with the ideas of many educational psychologists who focus upon how we learn and process information. My work at Curry College in the program that deals with learning disabilities has certainly re-inforced this. A few examples may help here. A child with poor eyesight will sometimes appear slow at learning. What has happened, in some instances, is that the child learned very early that seeing was *not* believing, and so stopped believing in eyesight. This could have the consequence that reading was avoided. Instead the child may have developed very impressive listening skills in an effort to get by. Such a person, in fact, may be a genius at sensing the overall importance of an idea, but completely helpless at working out the details, because he or she just 'can't see' them.

I give this example as just one of hundreds of examples in which the physical response to the outside world at an early age developed a series of behaviors that were designed to cope with the immediate need, and became fixed habits. The child, mentioned earlier, who refused to defecate did so because it seemed the only thing he *could* do to control the situation or change his mother's departure into her staying.

Again, the insecure person may well regress, in adulthood, to a 'safe' phase of life -- and a typically safe phase is the oral incorporative phase (A1). Compulsive eaters normally do not devour spicy or exotic foods, nor do they focus on food that takes a great deal of careful attention in order to eat it. Artichokes, roast quail, fish on the bone, and so on, rarely figure to any significant degree in compulsives' diets. The emphasis is almost always on the bland, on bulk, and preferably white or pale. Pasta, potatoes, rice, bread...and ice cream and milk. The safe blandness and the filling quantities are most important and, as one man said to me the preference is, "Anything that doesn't need a knife - better still, only a spoon!" This is a retreat to the level of mother's milk.

Look around. I'm sure you can find examples of people you know who are rather too emphatically at one stage or another on the chart. What about yourself? What do you like to eat? Do you find yourself anxious and uneasy when you are hungry? Possibly this is a throwback to a time when, as an infant, you were hungry and waiting to be fed -- and as you waited you cried. Your whole world was wrapped up in the timely delivery of food, and your world had just failed you. I sometimes wonder if the fast food phenomenon has as much to do with infantile drives as it does with the supposedly fast pace of modern life.

Here is another example. A young woman I worked with had developed an allergy to her mother's milk shortly after birth. It had taken several days to discover she was allergic to all milk. What do you think that did to her sense of trust? What do you think it may have felt like to her mother? Can one imagine being the mother, ready to love and breast feed, only to be rejected and then left with a screaming, terrified baby for several days, 24 hours a day? You may already be a parent. What did it feel like to have the newborn in the house? Did it make you think of your own infancy and your parents' lives at the time? Write about it if you can. How do Erikson's ideas fit with your own experience of children?

Let's continue this idea. Do you have trouble letting go of things? Do you store away momentos and become a "pack rat"? What sorts of things do you have trouble throwing away? Think back to your earliest memories. What was it like to be you? Now look at yourself, as your parents might have seen you then. Do you think they'd have seen the same issues? Take the time to write about your reaction to these questions and to this section.

Failed parenting in these early stages can be very damaging. Working from Erikson's plan we can deduce that poor parenting in the first nine months of life is likely to produce deep damage, even psychotic behavior. In a psychosis the outside world is seen as so threatening that the individual "decides" to have nothing to do with it, and chooses a different, fantasy world. Between the ages of about nine months and two years, when the child begins to learn autonomy, poor parenting can mean that the child never fully develops the idea of personal presence or effectiveness. This tends to manifest itself later in the behavior that says that nothing is the individual's fault. This is what is known as a character disorder and represents a failure of the individual to take any control of aspects of his or her life. I have met several people in my life, many of them in positions of authority, who seem to claim compulsively that it was not their fault that something happened. Be aware of such people. For some it is merely an evasion and an excuse. For others it represents a genuine blindness. One young man I worked with decided to steal my car. I walked into the parking lot just in time to see him ram it into a tree. When I demanded, somewhat angrily, to know what he was doing he replied that my car was so easy to steal that he shouldn't be blamed for it. Still angry, I pointed to the damaged hood and before I could say any more he said, "That's your fault. Your brakes are no good." These were not mere wisecracking excuses, I have to say. The young man was so convinced that it was all my fault that he immediately offered to fight me about it, because *I* had got *him* into trouble! He really could not see that he had any responsibility in this at all. Luckily, I knew about his history of physical and emotional neglect since birth, and I was not tempted to fight him.

If the child has been fairly well grounded in a nurturing and warm reality, at least for the first two years, then any disturbance that may occur after that is probably likely to produce only neurotic aftershocks. Naturally, if the experience is profoundly shattering, then any amount of regression is possible, but it is not always likely. Good foundations, once laid, are hard to shake.

It should come as no surprise to us that Erikson's diagram raises almost as many doubts as it does certainties. In particular, his approach has been criticized because he seems to give inadequate emphasis to the way girls develop. As I write, the field of women's psychology is producing both interesting critiques of the heavily male-dominated field that psychiatry and psychology have become, and developing its own ideas. I will briefly give an overview of the material so that you can apply this information to your own experience.

Carol Gilligan's *In A Different Voice* (1982) analyzes the way women and men use conversation and demonstrates convincingly that women use conversation as a way of developing relationships, while men use it as a way of imparting information. Men, it seems, are much more likely to kill themselves for failures which affect their pride - such as business disasters - while women tend to kill themselves because of love or relationship problems. The language of being is remarkably different, as well as the uses of words.

Jean Baker Miller's *Towards A New Psychology of Women* (1976) analyses in some detail the plight of girls in school who, at about age 11, find themselves faced with male teachers and a male culture that does not prize intimacy, yet still tends to expect girls to be softer and more caring than boys. In order to preserve themselves in such a situation, some girls feel they have to be 'perfect' and yet because they are expected to be two things at once - competitive and caring - it is often easier to act dumb rather than risk criticism for excelling. The conflict can lead to self-doubt, panic, and eating disorders, and other symptoms including the 'breathy' voice (which is the opposite of authoritative) and the frequency of the response "I don't know" from age 14 onwards.

Deborah Tannen's *You Just Don't Understand: Men and Women in Conversation* adds to this and points out that men talk to 'score points' rather than to encourage sharing. In this situation an order can be interpreted very differently by the sexes. Men, it seems, have trouble taking orders because the implied subordination is perceived as threatening.

My own enquiries have bourne this out, and it seems that losing one's temper is perceived by men as a way of gaining control, while by women it is feared as losing control. Tears seem to work differently as well: for men public weeping is a sign of collapse, while for women it can frequently be seen as a sign of determination to resist. Certainly, neither functions exclusively in this way, and we have to be careful not to make too many blanket generalizations. Sorrow provokes tears in men and women alike and certainly when there is great mental anguish, collapse occurs in both sexes. I am relating tendencies within our Western Culture, as are the authors I have mentioned, which seems to imply that men and women really do speak in languages that are sufficiently different from each other. Think for a moment of an argument you have had with a person of the opposite sex. It can be a lover, a friend, a colleague, a relation - anyone. Try to see it from the other person's point of view based on the possibility that this new information may have some truth. Can you see that there may be a valid point made by the other person? If you can remain calm enough to think about this the ideas may be very interesting. Do you often feel that members of the opposite sex simply can't see you as who you are? What do you think women look for in men, or men in women? What do you want your spouse or life-

partner to value? What do you expect that person to forgive about you?
What rôle expectations do you think are forced upon you?

Men, it would seem, tend to feel they have to be the money-earners, and
in return, they expect to be able to blow that money in poker games, or 'toys'
such as cars, motorcycles, boats, guns, or however they wish. What are the
rewards you give yourself? How much of your resources (time, income,
personal space) do they absorb?

These are not idle speculations. In response to these questions some unusual answers can emerge. A man who wrote about this mentioned that he
restored vintage motorcycles as a hobby. Since he earned more than his
wife, he thought it was only reasonable he should be allowed the extra. In
fact, when he made a sober calculation, his hobby took up hundreds of
hours a year, his entire basement, and the family garage, while his den was
filled with books and magazines, spare parts, paints, and tools. And his
phone bills were astounding. When he calculated how much his hobby cost
him he came to the conclusion that it swallowed almost 25% of his annual
income. This not only made him a lesser contributor to the family finances
than he imagined, but it also made him aware that his wife put more money
into the family than he and claimed less 'rewards'. Yet the illusion persisted
of him as the breadwinner -- driving the larger car, expecting to have his
meals served, the house cleaned, and the children dealt with. Stunned by the
result of his investigation, the man realized he could simply buy already resurrected motorcycles far more cheaply than by doing it himself. Further
thought brought him to the conclusion that his hobby was his way of keeping something for himself in a marriage he felt had claimed too big a share
of his personal time. It was a passive rebellion hidden by the accepted rôles
society endorses. More alert to this now, he still restores machinery, but he
is careful to limit himself, spends far less time and money on it, and has
more fun with his extra cash - enjoying it with his wife, not in spite of her.

One could argue that he was at the Erikson anal stage at which hanging
on to things - the money, the machinery (which he refused to sell or part
with) was a way of reserving power and the illusion of control over a world
that was always changing. The vintage machinery was always 'past', a
'classic' item -- always beyond the normal conception of time. Machinery is
also a traditionally male area of expertise, and usually excludes women.
Talk to any woman who has taken her car to a garage recently and see how
she feels she was treated. Most of the time, if the garage is not a deperson-
alized muffler or brake place, women report being treated kindly but as if

they were not very bright. My point is simply that the man regressed in his hobby to 'save' himself part of what he feared he might lose in his marriage, his 'maleness' and the identity that involved, and that he 'held on' in ways that suggested a very primitive response based in the first years of life. The *response* was to take the feeling that could be traced back to the anal stage and act it out in a way that was socially acceptable for a 40 year old male living in the U.S. middle class. The feeling had found its language. Unfortunately, by giving in to the feeling he had almost managed to wreck his marriage and his finances.

Erikson is not perfect. No theorist ever is. But he's provided a few insights, I think, that we would rather have than not. I've mentioned him in full awareness of the fact that he does not seem to deal with female sexual development very thoroughly. But that should be a good reason for you to discuss his ideas further in your own writing.

In this section we've spent a great deal of time covering a lot of material. The suggestions for writing explorations should help you to look further into these ideas. You will notice that the exercises are becoming a little less "organized" at this point, and that is simply because the very personal nature of the questions may make it hard for those in groups to share what they write. This should make no difference to you - you still have to explore these topics in writing.

CHAPTER THIRTEEN

I n this section I want to talk about sex and love.
Ironically, schools rarely teach us about love - at least not in class.
We will all fall in love, most of us several times in our lives, and yet there is
almost no formal training to tell us what to expect or how to avoid pitfalls.
Not surprisingly, everyone has a million sad tales, and very few good ones.

Do you find yourself dating the same sorts of misfits, losers and problem
people, over and over? Most of us do. The only way to break the pattern
for a better life is to ask why these people keep attracting you, and you
them.

You see, our sexual attitudes will have a lot to do with our early years.
Most of us will form ideas of maleness and femaleness that depend on the
parents or adult rôle models we observe and see praised. The sad cliché
about the ghetto child who wants to be like the neighborhood drug-dealer,
pimp or gang member is not only true, but true because the child sees who
has respect and power accorded to them, and plans to live accordingly.

Again, the Italian traditional families in my town remained that way generation after generation because children grew up with a strong sense of
what is correct within the family and tended to conform. In the age of equal
rights it seems astonishing that a man should expect his wife to stay at home
and raise children only, yet that is exactly what many of my fellow townspeople want -- and get. Sometimes there is rebellion and a child chooses to
live differently, but he or she may finally revert to the traditional pattern
even so.

My point is simple: for heterosexuals, the sexual partners we are going
to be attracted to are likely to be those who either (1) resemble our opposite

sex parent, in some way, or (2) who are the exact opposite of our opposite sex parent, if we do not have a good relationship with that parent.

In the case of homosexuality the modeling is a little more complicated, but we can generalize and say there are men who take on more feminine rôles in their relationships, and women who take on more masculine rôles, or who actually switch from one rôle to another, within the same relationship and depending on the rôle of the lover.

What needs to be said here is that people, whatever their sexual orientation and preference, tend to arrange things so they get what they *recognize* and *need*. The way they identify these needs is by comparison with internalized images of rôle models. These are very frequently parents. I'll give a simple example. If one finds oneself in a foreign country one tends to judge it by the standards of home. So we will often buy food that looks like what we expect food to look like, as we understand it. This may not be a good idea, in fact, depending on where you are. What looks like a piece of roast chicken in Peru may turn out to be guinea-pig, and full of unsavory parasites, possibly. A Madras version of a hamburger may look the same, but may well turn out to be very strange indeed because Hindu belief forbids the eating of beef. Part of the success of chains such as Macdonald's hinges on the fact that it is exactly the same item, at the same price, wherever one goes in the U.S. This is a way of saying that if we play safe with our food, preferring the familiar, then we are likely to play safe with our choice of partner. We go for what we know, whether or not what we know is what may be best for us.

This should not come as any surprise. We've all gone into stores looking for a certain item - furniture, clothes, whatever - and we've been unable to explain what we want, until we see it. Sometimes this works well, sometimes less so. A man I know has a mania for trying on and buying hats. Everyone who knows him thinks he looks dreadful in these hats, but he keeps buying them, convinced it makes him look dashing and handsome. Where he got this idea is unknown. The TV possibly? But no one can talk him out of the image of what he thinks he should be.

Again, two brothers I worked with both grew up in different ways to mirror their parents. Their father had been in the services and had moved the family around the world for years. The elder son joined an international organization, and the effect on him of his job was that he exactly replicated his father's lifestyle. He moved his family around the world at the request of his employers, every few years. The younger son became a college teacher and moved with each new appointment to a new neighborhood, or country. When each brother married they both married well-educated and self-assertive women, both of whose mothers had been killed during their early adolescence. Since each of the men had a rootless lifestyle, it meant that neither of their spouses could follow a career, which is exactly what the father's life had meant for their mother. As I began to explore this further, it also became apparent that neither daughter-in-law got on well with the mother (despite their obvious similarities) and that there had been some unpleasant arguments. It was as though the men had found women who would do the arguing for them. Both men admitted to evading the issue of challenging their mother, and both admitted that they were relieved their spouses' mothers were not alive. "Dealing with my own mother's bad enough, let alone with the 'mother-in-law' you see in sitcoms!" said one.

I give this example because it shows very strongly how family modeling can work. Each son replicated, in general terms, the father's life and values -- the job came before the family. The sons also repeated the father's choice of spouse, marrying someone who was prepared to give up career and family ties. In response to their mother's perceived faults, though, they both married not someone who was less-assertive (which would seem logical) but more assertive. Then they stood back and watched their wives make the break with the mother that they had never been able to achieve. The brothers had almost no realization of what this was all about, until they began to talk about it.

The exercise is, therefore, as follows: think of who your main parental rôle models are or were. Your real parents will be in there, but so, also, might your grandparents, an uncle or aunt. On a sheet of paper draw two vertical lines, to make three columns. Make a list of what you take to be the characteristics of the ideal man. This will be the 'male' page. The attributes can be both physical and mental. Now, on a new sheet of paper divided the same way, make a list of what you take to be the necessary attributes of the ideal woman. This will be the 'female' page. In the next column write down attributes that you see in your parent or role model of the same sex, and then (on the appropriate sheet) of the opposite sex. In the last column of the gender appropriate page write your own attributes. In the last remaining column note the attributes of a significant partner, either past or present. Looking at this list ask yourself where you got your idea of what a man was, and what a woman was? Now write them down.

When you have done that you may need to look very closely at the next part of the exercise. Who am I attracted to, and why? Since one is often attracted to many different sorts of people, we could narrow this down a little more. Who are the people with whom you have (or have had) complicated, difficult, *strong* relationships? Do you tend to be well-treated or badly-treated by these people?

What similarities or contrasts could you draw between these people and your parents? I always find it astonishing to discover how many people choose partners who have similarities to the opposite sex parent, even when the original parental relationship was not easy.

This, I should point out, is not an easy exercise. One may need someone to test ideas against, since it is often very difficult to see the patterns one is in. When I am working with a group this often means that I have to make extensive suggestions before the individual can begin to consider possible connections. For other people it works right away. One young woman, shattered by a disastrous love affair, couldn't understand why she kept forming relationships with men who had secrets and hidden compulsions, such as gambling, and who ultimately said they couldn't deal with her. As we looked further we discovered that her father had idolized her as a little girl. He was a minister but he fell in love with a parishioner and after a difficult divorce had to move away, abandoning his daughter. What she had learned from her Father, it would seem, was that men were creatures who made her feel very special, but that they had some hidden agenda, some personal strife, that made them abandon her. Certainly it cannot be easy for a minister to struggle with his emotions, with his belief and his family, and the young woman seemed to have had imprinted on her psyche at a very early stage that *men were preoccupied*. Sure enough, she chose relationships with men who were so preoccupied with their own concerns that they had little time for her - or only in bursts. When her boyfriend left her she felt a re-emergence of the same pain her father had inflicted. As a child her thought was that she could make her father "better". After all, he was always happy when he was with her - as far as she could see. In later life she refused to believe that she could not make her boyfriends "better" as well. As I've said in this book before, no one can make anyone else well. Only the individual can help him or herself.

The young woman's hope, as far as I can tell, was that she would be able to make one of these damaged souls well again, one day, and that this would compensate for her failure to do so with her father. The only trouble was that whenever she failed she could not look at the event and see that she had made a mistake with one person. Instead she would see in that failure all the people she had been unsuccessful with, including her father. This is a little like accidentally dropping a teacup and then, instead of sweeping up, remembering every piece of placeware one has ever chipped or broken. Seen like this, very few of us could ever feel good about our hand-eye coordination again! And yet who hasn't felt that? One knocks over the salt at an important public function, and who hasn't cursed themselves for a clumsy fool? A relationship falls apart and we've all felt the despair it brings, and the sense of self-doubt in those words that pass thorough our minds: "there must be something wrong with me."

Well, there probably *is* something wrong with you. There's something amiss with almost all of us. The danger lies in shaking one's head and feeling gloomy rather than searching for a way to stop repeating the same old mistakes. Guilt, "it's my fault," and blame, "it's their fault" are wonderful ways of avoiding coming to terms with the important task of getting things right.

Here is another very personal exercise. Usually I have group members do this and keep their public responses either general or let them remain silent. The reason will become obvious.

Think about your first love affair - your first real love that became sexual and that was an actual affair. A brief fling may have been exciting and romantic, and probably that is what you will write about anyway, but I'd like, if possible for you to think of your first love affair that you were able to treat as a relationship that had the possibility of a future. How did you first encounter each other? When was the first kiss? When you have visualized the memory, really felt it rather than seeing it through rose-colored glasses, think of how your intimacy grew. And now think about the physical act of sex, of lovemaking. Write about that.

Naturally, this is a very difficult topic to share, and so I suggest that you do *not* share it. The power of this exercise lies in the fact that whatever the course of our first real love affair, that is the pattern we are likely to repeat. Beyond this, whatever our pattern of sexual response that emerged, that, too, is very likely to be the repeated way our inner dramas are acted out. Now, before you become all upset here, please bear in mind that the first sexual experience is not what I am talking about. Most people's experience of sex is, at first, rather confused. What I am referring to is the way one responded sexually over time in this relationship.

I'll give an example. A man came to me because he was having difficulty with his lover. He wanted to make love more often than she, and he felt rejected and undervalued, while she felt objectified and used. Going back to his first love affair and examining it in detail allowed the man to gain a calmer perspective on himself and the loaded issue of sexuality, and to draw some valuable distinctions. The son of a dominant mother, he had chosen to pursue a strong-willed woman whom he literally had to persuade into bed, a pursuit that took a long time and a lot of energy. Since he had no sisters, his only close relationship with a woman had been with his mother, so it did not seem strange to him to have to persuade his lover into bed. After all, he'd always had to argue with his mother, so this seemed quite natural. The relationship developed with him doing all the pursuing, too. He remembered the affair as one in which he was always eager to make love, usually climaxed very quickly, and then had to work to get his partner to orgasm. It was nearly fifteen years later before he discovered he didn't necessarily always have to climax either a long time before or some time after his partner's orgasms. In conversations he revealed that from that very early time he had always assumed that he had to *give* pleasure. He therefore had tried hard and spent hours reading massage manuals so that he could be sure he gave pleasure. However, the problem was that he found it hard to *receive* pleasure. Intercourse was so overwhelming to him as a way to receive that he always climaxed very early, and then immediately felt he had to give pleasure to his partner. As a result of this, his partner was denied the joy of giving and the intimacy that can grow when giving and receiving is reciprocated. The man was so eager to be an adequate provider of pleasure that he forgot what he was feeling. Not surprisingly, intimacy died a slow but sure death.

What I want to extract from this sad case history is the fact that the pattern had been there from the very first - from the relationship with the mother - and that his first love set up a pattern of behavior that he repeated for fifteen years, until he took stock of the situation. Once he had identified the pattern, he began to see its absurdity. He relaxed. He began to do what he felt like rather than what he felt he had to. His sex and love life became far richer as a result. The last time we spoke he was also feeling more personally creative, as well.

It is, naturally, difficult to give statistical support to the validity of this exercise, and on the whole literature does not seem to deal with this in detail, the one possible exception being D.H. Lawrence. Lately some women writers have suggested this also - Terry McMillan comes to mind - but on the whole, it has been dealt with obliquely. An excellent example is in Shakespeare's *Romeo and Juliet*. If Shakespeare seems somewhat remote from us today, I apologise, but I feel the example is valid. When the lovers first meet they speak a perfect fourteen line sonnet. Each develops the other's images, each takes up the other's rhyme-scheme, and the exchange ends with their first kiss. This perfect balance of give and take is surely a suggestion as to the responsiveness each has to each intellectually, spiritually and sexually. I quote the whole section:

Romeo: If I profane with my unworthiest hand
           This holy shrine, the gentle sin is this:
           My lips, two blushing pilgrims, ready stand
           To smooth that rough touch with a tender kiss.

Juliet: Good pilgrim, you do wrong your hand too much
           Which mannerly devotion shows in this:
           For saints have hands that pilgrims hands do touch
           And palm to palm is holy palmers' kiss

Romeo: Have not saints lips, and holy palmers too?

Juliet: Ay, pilgrim, lips that they must use in prayer.

Romeo: O then, dear saint, let lips to what hands do.
           They pray: grant then, lest faith turn to despair.

Juliet: Saints do not move, though grant for prayer's sake.

Romeo: Then move not, while my prayer's effect I take.
                    [He kisses her] 1.V.92-105
                    (Arden Shakespeare)

The mutuality of these two lovers, who do in fact kill themselves for each other, is exceptional. Most of us will not find love quite so easy, alas, or so tragic, thank goodness. We will have to learn to love, and it may be a lifetime process, but we can help ourselves considerably if we identify early the sort of emotional confusion we may bring to the situation. Once we learn how to do something one way, it can be very hard to retrain.

If we consider *Romeo and Juliet* too clumsy an example let me give you something closer to home. We've all had the experience, or at least heard about it, of two people who meet and just 'click'. They laugh at the same things, like the same things, and seem to be miraculously in tune with each other from the start. These people are, in the same way as Shakespeare's pair, speaking the same language. Such mutuality bodes well for the rest of the relationship, although it is no cast iron guarantee of long term happiness. Even though a situation may start this way, how it continues should be the focus of our enquiry.

In this section I cannot give you any recipe for happiness in love. For one thing the section is very short, and miracles are hard to come by. All I can do is to urge you to look at how you do what you do, so that you can begin to discover why you do as you do. This may help you to change potentially poor behavior into something that can produce happiness. How much of your father or mother you have internalized will have a lot to do with this. This should be investigated in writing.

CHAPTER FOURTEEN

The topic of memory and how we remember things is a difficult one, since we always trim our memories a little - or a lot - almost as soon as the event is passed. "Someday we will look back on this too, and laugh!" The old saying tells us explicitly how we change distress into a funny story.

It seems likely that there are three levels to any distress. The first level is the feeling of distress. At that point each individual is alone in his or her private misery, and the tendency is not to share it, but to suffer. The second level occurs when the pain is relayed to another, and the third occurs when the events can be shared in a group, and defused. In a fascinating chapter in Jack Leedy's *Poetry Therapy* (Lippincott, Philadelphia, 1969) Dorothy Kobak relates her experiences working with disturbed boys. Once she had interested them in writing she noticed that they produced entirely different moods for different methods of writing. Their *poems* were melancholy, depressed and lonely, often with a sense of yearning for beauty. They did not want to share their poems. Their *short stories*, however, were adventure tales, hostile to authority and full of anger and violence, ready to be shared with others. When they came to write a *play*, they elected to work cooperatively and produced an irreverent and hilarious comedy. Ms Kobak suggested that the production of writing was a constructive act that appeared to give the boys great satisfaction, and that it became an avenue of permission that allowed them to join together as members of a group or society. I think there is much in this idea, but since Ms. Kobak doesn't quote the boys' work at length it is all rather theoretical.

My own experiences teaching writing to disturbed adolescents were similar, but I would like to use this to build on Ms. Kobak's ideas. The production of anything written was extremely threatening for the young adults I dealt with -- and it took quite an effort of encouragement before anything at all could be written. Initially the writing that did emerge was derivative and impersonal. Adapted popular music lyrics seemed to be very common. Gradually, there was a shift towards 'private' writing that sometimes was too personal to be shared. The personal writings were usually poetry, and usually somewhat obscure -- but the mood was always somber, introspective, and sad. It was very much as if the poetry was seen as the most personal of the ways to write, and I feel that here the young people were writing essentially to and for *themselves*. When they spoke about the poems, or wrote about them later, it was clear that in the awareness of an audience (of myself or of an imagined reader), the pain was less fully emphasized than the anger, and the chosen mode of communication was either one to one talking or brief stories or reminiscences. It was not until this stage had been reached that the experiences were ready to be shared in a larger group or written as a joint production, or even become impromptu dramatic performances. The mood of these productions was usually fairly hilarious and energetic. The pain that had once festered inside the individual found its way out and into laughter in this way. Within the hilarity I could usually note that the laughter had conquered the potential for depression and that the anger, instead of being smoldering and destructive, was now engaged in sarcasm, ridicule and even some good humor.

It seems to me that we have here three distinct phases in the externalization of pain, which we can name as (1) private, (2) inter-personal, (3) group shared. The private writing of pain is, as we have discussed, a form of naming, but when the pain becomes a shared topic, in phase (2) it is as though the individual is checking that the feelings are valid. "What!" cried one girl as she spoke tearfully to another, "you mean your Dad did that to you too? And you wanted to kill him, I bet, didn't you?" It was a relief to both young people to realize that the anger they felt was quite rational and normal considering the way they had been treated. Once the pain has been accepted and openly acknowledged, group sharing is the next step towards being able to be free of it. The hilarity of the group sessions became in one sense not so much a sharing of misery as a show of strength, a mood that seemed to proclaim that the group members had survived the worst that could be thrown at them, and they refused to be victims again.

This is what can happen in group work. If you are working on your own, you can make it happen, too. The first 'poetic' mode of self-communication can be the stepping stone either to talking with a confidant or writing to a trusted friend. Remember, if you do not feel you can trust anyone, then the person you write for, the person who you want to read what you write and understand your words, is someone who exists in the future. That should not be an excuse for not writing for that reader. Once you have done this, you may well find it possible to talk with and write to others about the topic, in a more general way. Most story writers and novelists I have spoken with write for one person - usually imaginary - who is their perfect reader. The exception to this is various mass market writers who clearly want to appeal as widely as possible. This in turn, tends to dilute the really personal content of what they say to almost nil.

The exercise I'd like to do now is one I know has been done by Sam Keen and his various collaborators, including Joseph Campbell. I had been doing my version of it for several years before I heard of their approach, but we essentially agree on the way this exercise can be used, although Keen and Campbell tend to describe the outcome in different terms.

Here it is, then, and it is relatively simple.

Think back to when you were a young child, say between 5 and 10. Think of the house or apartment you lived in. Can you draw a plan of it? Do so.

The exercise usually takes about half an hour, and then I encourage group members to talk about the plans they have drawn. Often, in the course of explaining an item, people will remember things about their lives and families and extra time is essential to allow for exploration, questions, and so on.

I got the idea for his exercise from an architect I worked with who also taught at a local college. He told me that one of the first assignments he had his aspiring architects do was to draw a sketch plan of their bedrooms. He found that they nearly always made the bed either far too big, or far too small for an accurate scale drawing. The point was that the areas we tend to be most intimately concerned with - like beds - loom large in our considerations so we tend to draw them larger than they are. Architecture, he explained, has a great deal to do with proportions and even more to do with how we perceive those proportions.

In the plans drawn from memory of the person at 5 or 7 years old, the child's bedroom will be, usually, very large, and it will tend to be the place

at which the drawing starts. Corridors will seem very long, and places beyond the child's obvious concerns may be hazy, or tacked on vaguely.
"There was a sitting room somewhere downstairs, but we weren't allowed in
it, because it was the 'best' room, for company, only..." as one woman put it.
As the age gets closer to 10 years old, the relationships between places begin to have more significance.

How big was your room compared to the other bedrooms? Were you
favored by the size or placement of the room, or did you feel crammed into a
corner? What about your parents' or parent's bedroom? What about the
public rooms of the house?

The way the plans are drawn has a great deal to do with the way memories and power acted in the home. One woman drew a very detailed plan in
which every chair, table and plant had a set place, especially her father's
chair, which she called The Throne. As she talked about her plan she became more and more angry, saying, "I can't believe I never noticed this before!" The picture that emerged was of a silent father, on The Throne, and a
mother who had organized the house but forbade anyone to move anything
because 'father wouldn't like it.' Since he was always silent, no one ever
found out whether or not this was true, but an aura of fear kept everyone
and everything in the home static. The power politics here were certainly
something to look at, as well as the implications about what the parents' relationship with each other might have been.

One man found it very difficult to put his parents' bedroom into the plan.
"It has to fit in here, somewhere, I think," he said, as he scratched out lines
and re-drew them. The difficulty was clearly signaled when he realized he
had drawn a bed in every room except his parents' room. He was able to
explain his confusion by the fact that his parents had divorced, but for some
years before that his father had been working late at his desk and had not
wanted to wake the mother by coming to bed late. When the mother started
sleeping in the spare room, the father remained on the couch and the master
bedroom became a dressing room - and so the room had become a symbol of
this confused relationship, empty at the core. It was not surprising the poor
fellow couldn't draw it.

Another drawing, by a woman, showed the garden and very little of the
inside of the house. Asked about this, she rapidly sketched in a few lines
talking about how she'd been given the smallest, creepiest room, and how it
was unfair. One part of the sketch was very confusing, and so I asked her
about this, and she began to explain that it was a spare room that she hated,

and she began to weep. The room, it turned out, was the one in which her music tutor had molested her when she was 10. It was not surprising that she preferred to draw the garden, and found the rooms to be unpleasant. Her shift from the unpleasantness of the home to the freedom and unenclosed nature of the garden was an evasion. It waved a red flag to me that there was something going on in the household that needed to be asked about.

Sam Keen and Joseph Campbell used this exercise in two phases - the house as remembered at 4 years old and the house remembered at 10 years old. They were interested in looking for the empty or 'missing' spaces as indicators of what had been repressed. I have tried their approach and found a number of draw backs. Frequently people have lived in the same house during the years 4 and 10 and so the memories are updated fairly regularly. If the person is still living in the house at the time of the exercise, it is likely that the confusions of the four year old have been blotted out, or updated, and so are difficult to recapture. I find that in asking the group to choose a time, and think back, that often individuals can recapture the flavor and mood of a particularly important phase of existence. This can over-ride the problem of continued habitation. Asking the group to do this twice, for specific time periods, often simply does not work because the detachment necessary to think back and feel the time period cannot always be achieved so easily. If one asks the group to do the exercise on different days, the detachment can be achieved, but there is always a feeling of having done this before that can undermine the exercise.

What I want to emphasize here is that the spatial relationships in the drawings can say a great deal about how the individual perceives the relationships in the house. Does one sibling have a bigger or better room? How far distant is the parental bedroom? Does the distance drawn correspond to the plan - do all the rooms fit together? One man drew a long corridor leading to his parents' bedroom and then couldn't quite get the plan to fit. He *perceived* them as distant, whereas they were actually in the very next room. Once again we are asking about memories that seem innocent enough to give us a glimpse of the unconscious, of the repressed, and of the relationships that may never have been fully examined before.

When doing this exercise I usually like to suggest to people that they recall the home they lived in at about the age of eight or ten. I give a possible span of ages from five to ten just because some people seem to have moved a great deal in their lives. Since I am eager to have them sketch a house plan that means something to them, rather than demanding a feat of memory, I give some lee-way. Ideally the later age bracket should be used. The reason for this is that between the ages of eight and ten the child comes into his or her own sense of power. School has shown us by this time that there are lots of people out there in the world, and that not all are treated the same way. We start noticing who has what, and what is socially acceptable with the other children in the playground. We bring this knowledge home, and begin to ask why we have the small bedroom when a sibling has a larger one. This is the point at which we first become consciously aware of the politics of the home in the sense that some people seem to have more power and control more space than others. It is this perception that I am seeking to have you recapture. Naturally, if I had asked you to explain the power politics of your family I might have received some rather astonished replies. By having you draw the situation we can see what might never have been formally spelled out. I suspect that in the future I shall be asking people to bring home videos of events in their lives, and this will be another window into a past that is nearly forgotten. With the price of video cameras constantly falling, we can expect it to be more common.

Thinking along the same lines, I'll mention another example. A relative of mine sends videotapes to his parents instead of letters. The interesting thing there is that of all the hours of the kids' birthday parties and so on, he, their son, always holds the camera and so never appears in the film. Ask the obvious question, what's missing? He is. We are left with the sad realization that clearly this man does not want his parents to know how he is doing - or possibly does not know how he is. Either way, he hides behind the camera. The video seems to say, "this is communication" but the actuality of it is that he is absent. One could argue that his unconscious desire to hide has led him to a course of action that has convinced his conscious mind that he is being open and honest with his parents. The Unconscious can often outwit us in using our intelligence against ourselves to keep itself (the Unconscious) unexamined.

With the idea of memory again before us, think back to your earliest memory. Naturally it doesn't have to be provable as the earliest memory. What is important is that you believe it to be one of the very earliest things you remember. This may be something that you may need several days to think about, and you may come up with several memories. Some of them may be dreams. In one sense it does not matter if they are real or imagined, what matters is that they should feel true. Write them down.

Embedded in these memories will be important information about your childhood *as you perceived it*. My own earliest memory is of sitting outside with my mother and elder brother. My brother and mother are talking or playing, but I am at a little distance, gathering daisies. Possibly they are making a daisy chain. The sky is full of dark clouds, and it will rain soon. I am perhaps 2 or 3 years old. When I began to examine the dream-memory I saw immediately that my mother's close, loving and possessive relationship with my brother was dramatized before me. While I was toddling about grabbing daisies, they were involved in a more intimate sharing. This has been a major dynamic in our family all our lives - sometimes very happily, sometimes less so. In this memory is the seed of important information.

I give my own example here because this exercise has taken me several years to complete, and I have been unable to test the memories of other group members in the same way. Certainly, if we look through literature we see the first memory as being an essential prefiguring of the life that follows. I think here of Virginia Woolf's *A Sketch of the Past* which begins:

I begin: the first memory.

This was of red and purple flowers on a back ground - my mother's dress; and she was sitting either in a train or on an omnibus, and I was on her lap.   (Norton Anthology. p. 1990)

Notice the intimacy of the memory, and the colors it involves - one does not remember such details out of idleness but because they mean something. Virginia Woolf acknowledges the fact implicitly and goes on to describe other memories that also were important in her life, showing what made her as she was, in her view. Freud felt that the earliest memory held important insights, too; and that is why we should allow our minds to roam backwards.

At this point I feel I should add one more thought. If, in the pursuit of these exercises, you find that the considering of these ideas is more than you can bear, stop. Get the professional help of a therapist. This is not to say that this book has failed you. It hasn't. But there are some things that it cannot do as effectively as you may need. Visiting a therapist will help you get to the bottom of specific concerns much more quickly. This book will have forced the door open, but your journey to mental wholeness will be much faster if you use the book in conjunction with a therapist.

CHAPTER FIFTEEN

I'm now going to do something rather different. I'd like to talk about art and doodles and about painting. We all know that famous artists have certain stylistic traits that mark their work. If this were not the case we would not be able to tell whether we were looking at a Rembrandt or a Picasso. What I would like to suggest is that all of us, great artists or rank amateurs, have our own styles that we bring to our sketches, doodles and cartoons, and that we tend to repeat certain patterns. This goes deeper than just the subject matter - although the subject matter is certainly a very useful clue to what the individual is thinking. If someone draws a picture of a person weeping it is a fairly good indicator that grief may be an issue, and needing expression. What I'm concerned with here is something a little different, namely, how to understand pictures that might not have an obvious emotional content. Here are some paintings I noticed at a friend's house some years ago. The paintings had all been produced by the mother of the owner. I was fascinated by them. Although they are all different, I was struck by certain underlying similarities. Take a look at them. The first page shows the paintings as they appear on the wall, the second page shows them with annotations designed to show repeated compositional elements.

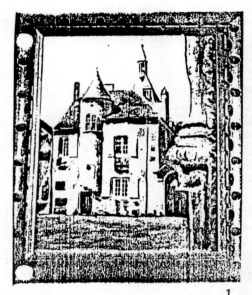

2

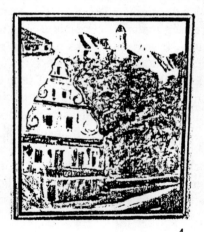

1

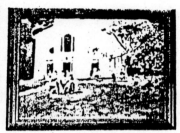

3

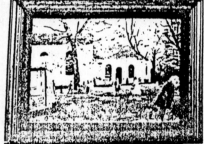

4

a

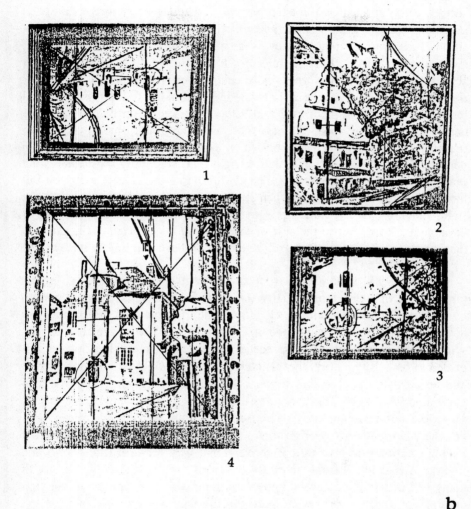

1

2

3

4

b

I then set about analyzing the paintings what I discovered didn't surprise me, although the clarity of these examples did. First, I drew two diagonals across each picture to find the center. In each case the lines intersected at a window/door or, in number 1, at a mysterious black smudge. This was the center of the picture. Then I traced the vertical axes of the pictures. There seemed to be at least two in each picture. In addition, picture 4 had been painted peeping around a pillar, while pictures 2 and 3 implied from the position of the branches that the view was similarly limited to the right hand of the picture by a tree. Each picture also has a curved diagonal line that cut across the top right hand corner. Also each picture has an important item at the place where the left vertical axis and the bottom left to top right diagonal intersects with it. In pictures 2 and 3 the item is a group of people. In 1 and 4 it is a large door. Doors; these are important, since they are so prominent. The eye seems to be led in each picture to the doors, but in number 1 it is the road running left to right that is actually most interesting (and more clearly emphasized). The church doors in 2 and 3 are open but blocked by figures. The real open ground seems to be in front and to the right, moving past the buildings. In picture 4 the door to this fortress is ominously closed, but to the side of the building, to the right, is a gateway that seems to offer a way forward. I've marked these exit lines with arrows.

I know very little about the artist, but it seems to me that what is important here is that this is essentially the same picture painted four times in terms of underlying structures. It is possible to argue that the painter had no idea this was happening, and it is equally valid to argue that unconsciously the painter chose those scenes because the internal structures appealed to her. Either way, the structures exist. I would go one step further and argue that the essential drama of the pictures lies in the problem of doors and windows. The doors are blocked, or closed, but there is a way forward around the houses. The houses are all old, venerable and imposing, but the road leads away from them. Could it be a question of the artist having to choose to give up the conventional way forward (the doors) and find her own route outside the established structure? The phallic quality of many of the details of towers, spires and long windows would suggest sexual content, that possibly what stands in the way is some idea of male expectation of what the painter should be. With this in mind, I called the owners of the pictures, Joan Goodman and Keith Goldsmith, for some details. They kindly agreed to give permission to reproduce them here.
The pictures had been painted by Joan's mother. The background to them is that the painter had been a very enthusiastic artist in her twenties and had then given up art altogether until the age of seventy, when she produced these beautiful canvases. The two church scenes were of the dog-

wood festival in Fairfield, Connecticut, and the building with the spires had been seen in Avallon, France. The last picture had no traceable source other than that it was a real place. I want to emphasize here that these were all real places. It is one thing to keep repeating the same idealized or imagined scene, quite another when the same repetition is to be observed in scenes that are not obviously linked. In an idealized scene one would expect the same elements to recurr. What was remarkable to me was that this artist (for these are very accomplished paintings showing mastery of technique and excellent draghtsmanship) seemed to have repeated the structural elements as part of her response to the outside world - these replications appear to have been absolutely unconscious.

The second point I want to stress is that the artist had indeed been blocked in her art production, for nearly fifty years. I do not know why this was, but I could speculate that the all-absorbing task of raising a family would have been a factor. The arrows, leading to the right in my annotations, can be seen, now, as the escape route that the artist had allowed herself as she began to paint again, finally, after years of not being able to express herself in this way.

After I had shown these pictures to a class a young man brought me two of his photographs of which he was very proud. He gave them to me, and asked my comments. I reproduce them for you to see, and with his permission. The comments I made at the time, with which he agreed, were that these were basically the same picture in that both the sidewalk and the river - both things that go somewhere - were seemingly blocked. In one the bridge cuts off the view, in the other it is the sidewalk, on which the photographer is standing, that is cluttered. He had not realized until we spoke how similar the pictures were.

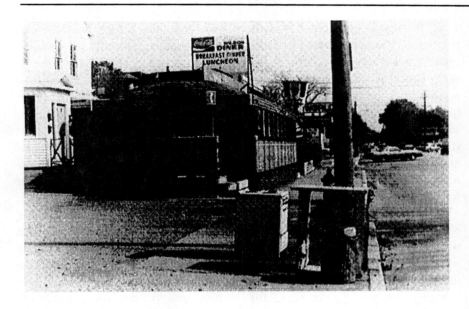

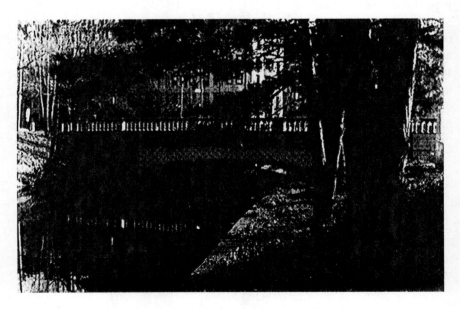

This personal drama had worked itself through in pictures rather than paintings. I suggested to this man that although the river and road seemed blocked, they were not in fact, and this is implicit in the pictures. There is a future, I suggested, even if at present it looks rather closed down. The progression from left to right (which is the same as in the paintings) is the natural progression of writing or reading. This would seem to imply that the unconscious, at least, believed that he was moving ahead. The slowness of the river compared with the stasis of the viewpoint of the other picture. Taken from the sidewalk it implied that the photographer was a pedestrian while the traffic rushed past behind where he stood. When he and I talked a little more, he confessed that he did feel that his personal progress was painfully slow, and that his emotions (the water element) were not enlivening or life-giving. One would not want to drink from the river in the picture, he agreed.

As I have worked with groups I have often come across examples that mirror these, but few were this clear and straightforward, which is why I am using them. My method of analyzing these pictures is not sophisticated, but it does, I believe, point out things that are undeniably present.

Sometimes these patterns are very consciously present, but severely repressed. I show here some pictures taken from the case files of a doctor treating a young woman for psychiatric disturbances in about 1915. The doctor preserved the pictures, some of them careful paintings, some sketches, as part of his notes.

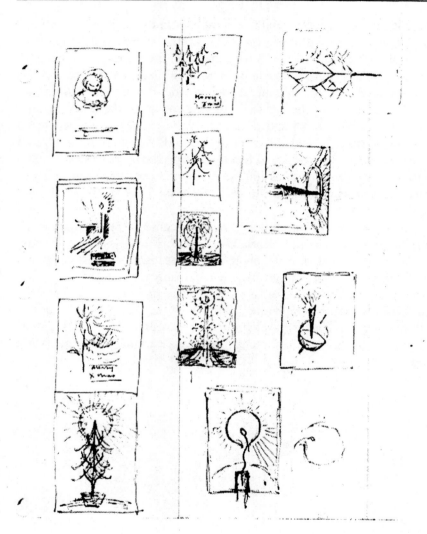

a

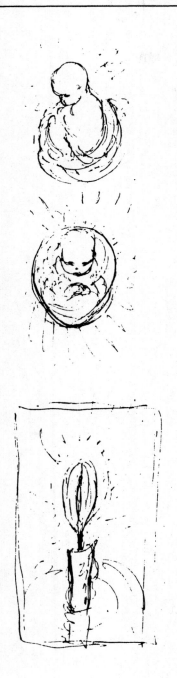

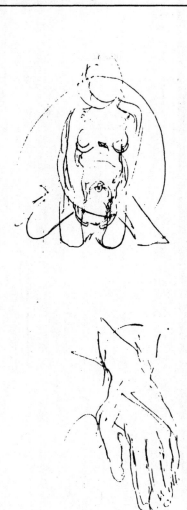

b

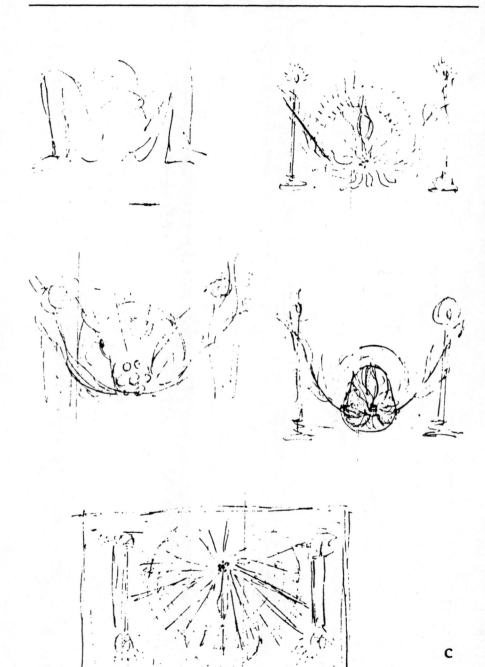

c

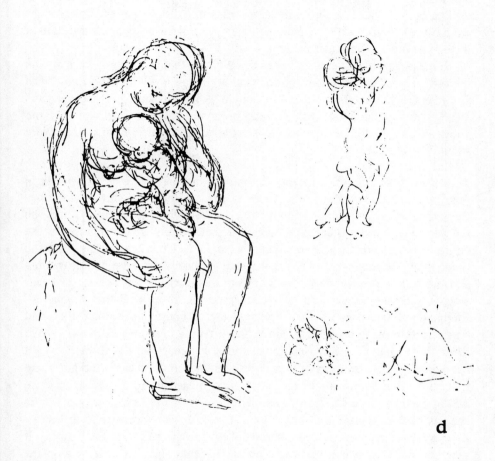

d

I would like to direct you to the Christmas card designs (A) and then to the second series of designs (B). Christmas is, of course, the celebration of the birth of Christ, and we notice in (B) a sketch of a woman giving birth and of a candle with a flame like a vagina. In (C) the birth sequence is quickly disguised as two candles and a bright something or other on an altar. As we look at (D) we notice the conventional mother and child and then two sets of figures that seem to be copulating. Turning back to (A) now we can identify candles, which seem phallic but which have vaginal flames - a variant being a 'star' on top of the Christmas tree design - and at lower right we have what is clearly a candle producing a sperm at its wick that enters the egg of the candle's aura of light.

Some of the other notes and sketches indicate that this young woman was not only a good artist, but was receiving a college level education, and was intelligent and analytic. What I wish to point out here is that she was clearly very preoccupied with sex and pregnancy at this time, and that she knowingly repeated the same patterns yet tried to disguise them so they were socially acceptable.

I offer these examples to you so that you can be aware of tendencies in your own art, and in that produced by others. After I had shown these pictures to a group, a young woman came to talk with me privately, and she showed me her latest piece of art which depicted a lily flower in a circle, the entire effect of which was to suggest a vagina. I mentioned this, and she immediately began to explain that this was precisely why she had drawn it - and she had worked on various versions of this drawing for weeks. The reason she did so emerged in a later conversation. It appears that a year beforehand she had found herself pregnant and although she wanted the child was afraid to bring it to term. Since that time she had been in mourning for the child she had not had. Her sense of loss, her fear that the abortion might have damaged her chances of becoming a mother in the future, and her sense that something beautiful (love making) had turned into an ugly experience all emerged in the picture that she gave me. In it the female genitals were seen as fresh and pure and flower like. It was a wish to return to an earlier time and also an assertion that she would renew herself, like the flower. It was not until she was able to talk about this that she was able to stop the obsessive re-drawing of the image. Until she found the language to say what she meant, the flower *was* the language.

What does this mean for you, you may ask? I think that what it shows is that in our repeated behavior patterns, of which this is merely another example, we dramatize our own feelings. The expression is both a statement of what we feel, and a disguise that is asking to be de-coded. And this brings us to our exercise.

Think of someone who interests you. Now, what are the questions you want to ask that person? What are the things you are afraid to ask that person? Write down several. Thinking now of yourself, what are the questions that you would *like* someone to ask you? What are the things that you consider that someone *should* ask you? What is it that you are *afraid* someone will ask you?

Take the time, now, to write answers to all these questions.

Whether you are alone or in a group it will be difficult to share some of these replies. In my view each of us radiates things that we want to be questioned about. It may be simply something like: "where did you buy those shoes?" That will enable us to talk about the great bargain we snapped up. Usually it is a little more than this. In this way we engage people in our concerns in a very controlled way. I would suggest, though, that there are many things that we know we should be looking at in our lives that we try to convince ourselves are just fine. Those are the things we are afraid to be asked, although ironically enough, I believe we are actually more afraid that we will *not* be asked. One man I knew emerged from his first session of therapy with a broad grin and announced, "They didn't get a thing out of me!" Yet he had gone there voluntarily. He really wanted to be asked about his pain, (that was why he had gone) but he was afraid to have to talk about it. I suspect that he's not a rare case.

Since then I have come across a man who has visited eight marriage counselors with his wife, and each time, after one session, he leaves and finds a new counselor. He claims that each one is "not right" for him... Again, a woman I observed for a time went to her first counseling session in a year and stormed out after two minutes because the counselor asked how she was doing with her drug problem. "That's got nothing to do with it!" she screamed as she left. But of course, it had. There are, you see, a million disguises. But we, each one of us, know exactly what it is we are afraid to be asked about. Possibly we should be asking ourselves these questions...?

Write about it.

To this we can add another exercise. This one came to me as I was sitting in my favorite Chinese restaurant, and I was so disappointed with the fortune cookie fortune I received that my companions and I immediately set about making more exciting fortunes. We had a lot of fun with this. So here's the exercise.

Write two fortunes you would like to receive.
Write two fortunes you would like to send to a parent.
Write two you would like to send to a loved one.
If you could place a free gift in packets of breakfast cereal, what would it be?

The results are invariably amusing, at the start, expressing wishes and desires - hopes for the future. This is healthy, it seems to me, because too often we confine ourselves to the possibilities of here and now, and we do not have much chance to exercise our fantasies. Fantasy can alert us to bigger possibilities for our lives. A fortune that read, "you will go to a Caribbean island and open a fabulously successful movie house" summed up precisely the desires of one young man who wanted very much to do something different with his life, but felt he couldn't. Although he didn't fulfill the fortune to the letter, writing it down and sharing it enabled him to get supportive reactions from the group. They all thought it was a great idea. Energized by this, that young man has made several major changes in his life. At the time he wrote the fortune, however, he thought that any change at all was impossible.

The fortunes written for the parents, I find, are usually balanced between statements of appreciation and statements of advice. "Your children love you more than you realize," wrote one woman. With those very few words she was able to describe the central tension in her family, a tension she was later able to write about. "Give up the booze, Dad. It's killing us all," wrote a young man. In that short pair of sentences he was able to inform the group about a major concern in his life, and deliver a message he was afraid to say directly to his father. In so doing he was able to acknowledge his pain and see, for the first time, that he was not to blame for it.

The fortune directed to a loved one often allows the writer to say tender or challenging things that cannot be said to the person directly. These are as varied as the people who write them, but one that will always stick out in my memory is the one directed by a woman to her lover which read, "let someone else win, sometimes." The competitive and argumentative side of the lover was certainly at issue here, and writing this allowed the woman to explore the topic in greater depth, so she could discuss it in a controlled way, later, with her lover. It gave her a chance to examine and smooth out a potentially difficult concern in her relationship, when simply talking about it to the group would have seemed too threatening.

The gift in the cereal box is always challenging, because the answers are very varied. "A Captain Crunch Compass!" declared one man in his mid-twenties, with a huge grin. It was, he maintained, the best toy he'd ever had in a cereal packet and it had transformed his summer at age eight. This then led him into a discussion of his childhood at that time, and this was an important issue since he was one of a family of ten, not counting several neighborhood children who he thought were his brothers but were actually his brothers' friends who did not get on with their own parents, and who had moved in for a few years. The discussion allowed him to consider what was 'his' in the family home, and to relive the excitement of independence, of finding his own way through the woods with the help of his trusty compass. The fortune he wrote brought back for him important memories of his childhood.

An older woman wanted to put condoms in packets of Cheerios, she said, "so no one has any excuse not to have safe sex". It took little prodding before she began to speak about her teenage daughters and her fears that they would get pregnant or contract AIDS. Although she had talked with her daughters about this she was not sure they had taken her words seriously, and she was very worried.

This is usually a light-hearted exercise, but one that can cut straight to the central issues, as you can see. Sometimes confining group members to brief sentences, such as fortune cookies usually supply, can enable them to focus on what is most meaningful to them at that time, as well as encouraging them to think about their own futures, wishes, and dreams. I have tried the exercise in various forms, including the 'write your own horoscope' version, but that tends to make group members write at greater length and with less precision. The horoscope works best with a small group when there is plenty of time, while the fortune cookies are more effective in the larger group of ten or more. If you are working on your own, you may find it beneficial to do both.

What were your fortunes? How would you elaborate on them? If you are not happy with your initial responses, how would you change them? Why?

CHAPTER SIXTEEN

We are now approaching the end of our exercises and meditations on what the mind may do and how it may function. We do have a few tasks left, though, and they are best achieved through the re-assessment of all we have looked at so far. In other words, it's time to re-read all those exercises and the after-exercise thoughts they provoked. With luck you will have linked the exercises to your daily life, and have written about it. Did you keep a journal, as suggested? If so, what sort of journal was it? Was it different from other journals you may have kept? If you didn't keep a journal or notebook, why not? Are the reasons you give for not keeping it strictly true?

Here are some things to look for in your review of your work.

I. Are the exercises in the written form the same as your memories of them? You may have forgotten some, and others may seem to you to be almost miraculously subtle whereas they are in fact quite straightforward. Which ones did you forget? Why do you think you did so? Which ones worked for you? What did you discover? Do your memories of events in the rest of your life correspond, in re-reading, to what you wrote?

II. Did you ask any questions about yourself you could not answer at the time? Did you consider them in depth? Or did you forget them? The vocabulary of questioning in this way is always provisional, and will contain words and phrases like: possibly, I think, probably, it seems likely...and so on. This shows the ability of dealing with uncertainty, of dealing with questions that it may take a while to solve. This can be seen as a very mature adult trait. This is the adult part of your consciousness at work.

If, on the other hand, you find that there are few questions in your writing, and that the writing is loaded with wishes, desires and statements of confusion - "I don't know" and "I don't care" - then we are dealing with a part of the personality that is a little less mature. Similarly, extremes of vocabulary which occur in phases, as, for example - absolutely, unbelievably great, awesome, the best, the pits - these all come from a less than mature capacity to make judgment calls. One could call this the child part of the personality, or the Id.

The person who reviews his or her work and notices words like: should, ought, always, never, never again, once again, might like to be aware that these are all phrases and words that tend to be used judgmentally. Labeling people has the same effect, especially if the labels tend to diminish the complexity of the individual. This is the voice of the parent part of the personality, the Superego.

You will probably find all three 'voices' in your writing. Notice, though, when you tend to be in 'child' mode and when in 'parent' mode. Can you reassess each episode using 'adult' mode language?

III. Did you write about the present as well as the past? Where is the present in your writings? Do you dwell on the past? Where is the future? Another part of this is the idea of guilt. Do you feel guilty about the past? Guilt and self-blaming are usually a way of avoiding having to face the present situation. If one says, "I made a mistake" the rational thing to do is to avoid making that mistake again. There is no guilt, there. If one allows oneself to feel guilt that is roughly the same as saying, "I *am* a mistake." In this circumstance one has no duty to do differently in the future because one is helpless, hopeless and bound to mess up. The only way out of guilt is to take responsibility. Remember Orestes? Do you take responsibility for the actions you have recorded? An easy way to tell is to look for the occurrences of 'I'. Am 'I' in the record at all? Or are things being done to '*me*'? Where do you tend to use guilt and self blame? Is there a repeated pattern of any sort here?

IV.   Did you find that in the course of writing you revealed something of your own nature to yourself? Was the writing truly exploratory?

V. Did you record pleasant moments as well as painful ones? What do you think of yourself after all this? Do you see any personal strengths, here?

VI.   Did you take what you learned in the exercises and apply it to your life? It is eminently possible to write reams of complaint and exploration about one's siblings, parents, lover, spouse, whoever, and yet not reveal the feelings to the person most intimately concerned. Do you really want to heal this relationship? Do you believe it is possible? Or do you just want to complain about it? At what point does the complaint merely mask a reluctance to do anything? Do you *really* want to change? The unconscious is very good at misleading us here. By complaining to a diary or to a confidant we may temporarily cope with a feeling, while in actuality we are afraid to do anything about it, and we're ashamed to admit we're afraid. But complaining has given us the illusion that something has been done.

This brings us to the next major consideration -- do you really want change in your life? You can do all the exercises in the book, learn a lot about yourself and still not get around to changing your life. Like a smoker who knows how dangerous it is, but still goes ahead and smokes anyway, we are all capable of knowing what must be done but not feeling the need to change. We know with our brain, but feel with our hearts, after all.

There are many reasons for this, and I'll outline a few here. The first is habit. I'll give an example. I was with some colleagues, all of whom were mental health workers, and we were talking about our particular foibles and mild neuroses. One man worried continually that his car would break down, another needed to go home for a certain period each day or he felt he could not work effectively, and so on. Nothing too serious here, we decided. Then one of our circle said, half in jest, "Why don't we all borrow each other's neuroses for a few days?" There was laughter, jokes then silence. Finally one person spoke, and he really spoke for all, when he said, "But I like my neuroses. I've spent most of my life developing them. I'm not sure I want to give them away..." The point here is that we do grow to love our faults, sometimes. Take them away and we feel loss. Under these circumstances we're unlikely to change because we actually like our slight craziness. Please don't misunderstand. I'm not suggesting that we should all be reduced to a uniform greyish 'normalcy', nor that we should want to be. I'm using this as an example to show that often behavior is so much a part of the person that leaving it behind is a very threatening suggestion.

An acquaintance once hurt his leg and had to walk with a cane for a few weeks until the injury healed. He noticed that during that time he was treated with deference and that the stick actually made him more memorable to those with whom he was networking. He now uses a stick constantly and even limps occasionally, although there is nothing wrong with his leg, as he will freely admit.

The compensation undertaken here, to deal with physical discomfort, is exactly the same as what can happen with mental distress. Lord Byron's melancholy cannot have been much of a pleasure for him initially, yet it helped to boost his reputation as a poet and certainly enhanced his sex appeal. Who could blame him if he kept his mannerisms? And if he hadn't been successful, could he have borne to retain his gloom? The world of British Society wanted their poet to be like this, and so he obligingly became fixed there, in that behavior. The voluntary, or chosen reaction can become an end in itself so that the individual finds it very hard to change back.

I call these "obstacles to change", and there are several that can be identified, although all are linked. Here is a typical piece of behavior: a person is disappointed and depressed and decides to use alcohol to forget the problems. The problems do not go away, they are merely evaded for a brief time. Meanwhile, other problems emerge as alcohol threatens the stability of job, of marriage, of finances, and much more. Clearly the need is to change the behavior. Yet no change is forthcoming. What is getting in the way? Here are some suggestions:

1. *Fear*: Dealing with a problem can seem so frightening that it never is dealt with. A neighbor of mine, I discovered recently, died of breast cancer. I had known her very slightly - enough to nod good morning as we passed in the street. It appears that she was afraid of surgery and even more afraid of medical bills, since she had no health insurance. Although the cancer was diagnosed nearly two years earlier, which gave her an excellent chance of recovery, she did nothing. The first I knew of it was when the ambulance came, a week before her death. Naturally, I do not know her psychological state in detail, but I have to say that it's fair to deduce fear as a major aspect of her failure to act.

2. *Low self-esteem*: This I define as the belief that one really does not deserve to have a better or happier life, or even a life at all. It is surprisingly common. If one does not think that life can be happy, then one is likely to arrange a life that confirms the suspicion. When I was a student in Britain many of us were living rather less than luxurious existences on student grants. After a few years of drafty lodgings, poor diets, and cheap clothes, many of us began to think that poverty was our future, as well as our present. Unhappily, quite a few of my contemporaries began to believe it, and they have gone on to live their lives with diminished expectations -- and become proud of it, too. The fact remains, however, that better hous-

ing, food and clothing will help to ensure better health and longer life. I don't think many people would argue against these advantages for themselves or their families, but the feeling that one has no right to expect better can be very dangerous. It is very common and is often a result of schooling or family influences, but it can be overcome. Everyone has the right to be happy.

3. *Ignorance*: This comes directly out of point 2 above, and the belief that one is not deserving of good things. Since one does not believe that things can be better, a mental paralysis can descend in which one is quite simply unable to see any alternative course of action, and there is a likelihood of being left with no idea of what one wants. Take the example of a worker who is laid off. Such a person may have expected to be a worker all his or her life, doing only a certain type of work. As a result, the person may have a fixed image of him or her self, and instead of thinking in positive terms about what he or she could do, there is a greater likelihood of gloomy acceptance of redundancy and poverty. This ignorance often has nothing to do with the intelligence of the individual. I've seen IBM executives who could not think what to do once their job was gone, and had no idea what they felt like doing. I've also seen out-of-work janitors who put together a painting and decorating company, and had more work than they could handle. Ignorance means deliberately ignoring or choosing not to know, and we can all fall victim to it.

4. *Reasons not to Change*: This grows out of 3. We can all think of a million reasons not to change our lives, jobs, personal relationships. All of the reasons will seem to have some value. Many may be defensive; all of them will stop the process of change if they can. In my experience a reason does not even have to be good in order to prevent change. One woman remained in her marriage because she didn't want to split the photograph albums, which is the way she imagined the divorce proceedings. A man I worked with didn't want to leave his lover because of their dog. He was afraid it would pine for him. Sometimes the reasons are real, but have no validity. A family of four for years went to visit the grandmother and discovered only after her death that they had, all four, hated the way the visits developed. Each had been afraid of voicing his or her own doubts for fear of upsetting the others, who had all seemed happy with the relationship. The desire not to rock the boat is surely valid, but here it developed into a conspiracy of silence.

One of the biggest reasons for not changing is next.

5. *Lack of Help: and the failure to ask for it.* If you need help, ask. Very few of us can change our lives entirely on our own. That is at least one reason that led you to buy this book - to help you make a new future. If you really want to change you may need even more help: a friend, a therapist, a clinic, a program. If you need help, GET IT. I should know, because I used to be angry at all those people who should have *known* I needed help. They should have read my mind! They'd failed me! O.K., if that's the way it is, I'll never ask for help from them again! Or so I concluded.

The truth is that people are busy and few of them can read minds. So if you need help it really is up to you to overcome your resistance and get help. But be careful. The other side of this is to expect that everyone will immediately rush about and solve the problems, your problems. Well, people can be very helpful, of course, but often only with surface problems. A friend can loan money, but if you have a compulsive shopping problem, the money will not help you to control the behavior. If you need therapy, find a therapist. Even then, the therapist cannot sort out your mind for you; you have to work *with* the therapist.

Frequently people will look around and announce in despair that there's no one out there who can be relied upon - no one can help. This is hardly likely. At last count there were over five billion people in the world, and the thing that always astonishes me is how much wisdom, knowledge and understanding is often very close to hand. But it has to be sought out. This can be part of the next obstacle to change, also, which is perfectionism.

6. *Perfectionism:* I knew a man who went with his wife to nine marriage counselors and four therapists. He visited each one once and then moved on, announcing that this person was 'not right for them'. Needless to say, the marriage never did get the guidance it needed. His perfectionism was used as a way of avoiding the confrontation with the real problem.

Another form of perfectionism concerns housing. Two associates of mine visited over one hundred properties looking for a house to buy. Nothing could fit the bill because they wanted the house to have everything they wanted. They still have not bought a house. Sometimes if you wait for all the circumstances to be perfect, it's a little like waiting for the decision to be made for you. No house is ever completely perfect, no therapist is perfect. Only God can fulfill the rôle of perfection, presumably, and not necessarily then if one believes in the Greek and Roman myths.

Perfectionism also works the other way, in that the person who wishes to change cannot do so because it means taking the risk of failure. Wanting to be a poet is admirable, but refusing to be one because one can never be as good as Shakespeare is hardly sensible. To begin with, one is unlikely to know if one is going to be as good as Shakespeare until one has been a poet for some time. Some of Shakespeare's early plays weren't that great, and some are rarely played for that reason. *Titus Andromicus* is a curiosity by any standards, and *The Comedy of Errors* is so derivative that for all its good points, it would hardly be read today if it were not for Shakespeare's later works.

It takes real courage to risk change. The chances are that very few of us will become immediately famous because of our life changes. But that is not the point. The point is to become happier, more fulfilled, and more authentic to one's self. If we do not do that, then fame is a hollow reward.

Perfectionism can hold us back from everything because, quite simply, nothing and no one can ever measure up. Whether you apply perfectionism to yourself - 'I can't do X because I'll never be any good at it' or to another, 'I can't marry X because he/she is not perfect' or to the time itself, 'this is not the right time to do it' - the result is paralysis. We live in an imperfect world, and to wait for it to perfect itself for our purposes is a dangerous delusion.

The last obstacle to change that I want to mention is one that on the face of it seems to be no obstacle at all, and that is:

7. *Determination*: Determination is wonderful, and it will help you to make the first steps in change, but it is a two edged sword, and can leave us unprepared for the full demand the change puts on us. What does that mean? To explain I'll draw on the work of Dr. Emile Coué, the discoverer of the Coué method. What he expressed can be boiled down to roughly this: first, if the imagination and willpower are in conflict, imagination will always win, since it comes from the core of one's being. Second: imagination can be trained and developed, but we have to force ourselves to do things by willpower, and so we generate stress. Imagination, if properly used, reduces the stress level.

A simple illustration of this idea might be a man who wishes to give up smoking. He can will himself, through determination, to stop smoking, but he will still want to do it, and thus be under stress. A way around this is to work on the man's imagination so that he constructs an idea of smoking as damaging and nurtures an image of himself as free of cigarettes, saving money, becoming fitter and healthier. This image exists in the imaginative realm of the mind and makes the whole procedure of giving up easier. It counteracts the associations built up by the smoker over time. Part of the attraction of cigarettes, as we may well suppose, is the glamour of the act, as relayed to us in advertisements, and the mental pleasures of relaxation and friendship which are often associated with smoking. These exist in the imagination. Determination alone cannot beat this for very long. The result then is that the smoker returns to cigarettes with a feeling that this is a habit that cannot be broken, after all. Blind determination is never sufficient. One needs reasons that resonate in the imagination, and then one certainly needs determination, as well.

Reviewing these seven items, it is not difficult to see that they are inter-linked. Perfectionism (6)- the fear that nothing will come right if one changes - is only another version of what happens in cases of low self-esteem (2), where the expectation is that nothing will ever turn out well. Too much determination (7) may cause us not to ask for help (5), or we may ask the wrong people to help us because, at bottom, we do not believe in a successful outcome. In this way, we can easily sabotage ourselves. Fear (1) gives us a million reasons not to do anything, which is covered by (4), reasons not to change. Fear also makes us ignorant (3) despite our intelligence. All are interlinked. I have written them out like this in list formation not because they are separable, but merely to help you remind yourself about them, because we all need reminding from time to time.

This brings us to the end of our work together. By all means close the book and chat to your friends about all the good stuff that's in it, but please - don't talk about it and not live it. Apply what you've learned. Don't put it off until you've read a little more about it elsewhere. That's a version of perfectionism creeping in. 'I'm not ready yet.' If you think like that you'll never be ready, I suspect. All I can do is encourage you to move ahead. Remember, it's your life, not mine. Good Luck!

BIBLIOGRAPHY

Barthes, Roland	*Mythologies* (transl. Annette Lavers) St Albans: Paladin, 1972
Beattie, Melody	*Beyond Codependency*. San Francisco: Harper and Row, 1989
" "	*Codependent No More*. San Francisco: Harper and Row, 1987
Berger, John,	*Ways of Seeing*. Harmondsworth: Penguin, 1972
Birch, Alison Wyrley,	*Poetry for Peace of Mind*. New York: Doubleday, 1978
Bly, John	*Iron John*. Reading, MA: Addison-Wesley, 1990
Bolen, Jean Shinoda	*Goddesses in Everywoman*. New York: Harper and Row, 1984
" "	*Gods in Everyman.* New York: HarperCollins, 1990
Cameron, Julia	*The Artist's Way*. New York: Tarcher/Putnam, 1992
Erikson, Erik	*Identity*. London: Faber, 1968
" "	*Childhood and Society*. St Alban's, Paladin, 1977
Freud, Sigmund	*On The Interpretation of Dreams*. (widely reprinted)
" "	*The Psychopathology of Everyday Life*. (widely reprinted)
Goldberg, Natalie	*Wild Mind: Living With the Writer's Life*. New York: Bantam, 1990

" "	*Writing Down the Bones.* Boston: Shambhala, 1986
Gilligan, Carol	*A Different Voice.* Cambridge, Harvard Univ. Press, 1982
Holland, Norman	*Poems in Persons.* New York: Norton, 1975
	Journal of Poetry Therapy. Human Services Press.
Jung C.G.	*Man and His Symbols.* New York: Doubleday, 1964
Kaminsky, Marc	*What's Inside You It Shines Out Of You.* New York: Horizon, 1974
Koch, Kenneth	*I Never Told Anybody.* New York: Random House, 1977
" "	*Rose, Where Did You Get That Red?* New York: Random House, 1973
" "	*Wishes, Lies, and Dreams.* New York: Chelsea House, 1970
Kubler-Ross, Elisabeth	*On Death and Dying.* New York: Macmillan, 1991
Laing, R. D.	*The Divided Self.* Harmondsworth: Penguin, 1962: Reprint Pelican,1974
" "	*Self and Others.* Harmondsworth: Penguin, 1961: Reprint Pelican, 1971
" " & Esterson, A	*Family, Madness, and Society.* Harmondsworth: Penguin, 1961
Lee, John	*Writing from the Body.* New York: St.Martin's, 1994
Leedy, J. J. (Ed.)	*Poetry Therapy.* Philadelphia: Lippincott, 1969
" "	*Poetry the Healer.* Philadelphia: Lippincott, 1973
Leonard, Linda S.	*On The Way to the Wedding.* Boston. Shambhala, 1986
" "	*The Wounded Woman.* Boston,: Shambhala, 1983
Lerner, Arthur (Ed.)	*Poetry in the Therapeutic Experience.* New York: Pergamon,1973
Marks, Robert (Ed.)	*Great Ideas in Psychology.* New York: Bantam 1966
Moody, M.&	*Bibliotherapy Methods and Materials.* Chicago:

Limper, H.K.   American Library Association, 1971
Miller, Alice   *The Drama of the Gifted Child.* New York: Basic
                         Books, 1981
   "   "   *Thou Shalt Not be Aware.* New York: Meridian,
                         1986
Miller, Jean Baker   *Towards A New Psychology of Women.* Boston:
                         Beacon Press,1986
Peck, M. Scott   *The Road Less Traveled.* New York: Simon and
                         Schuster, 1978
Pipher, Mary   *Reviving Ophelia.* New York, Ballantine, 1994
Pinkola Estes, Clarissa *Women Who Run with the Wolves.* New York:
                         Ballantine, 1992
Rainer, Tristine   *The New Diary.* Los Angeles: Tarcher, 1978
Rogers, Carl   "Empathic: An Unappreciated Way of Being"
                         The Counseling Psychologist vol.5, no.2 1975
Schloss, Gilbert A.   *Psychopoetry.* New York: Grosset and Dunlap,
                         1976
Simon, Sidney   *Getting Unstuck.* New York: Time Warner,1989
Steinem, Gloria   *Revolution From Within.* Boston,: Littlebrown,
                         1992
Tannen, Deborah   *You Just Don't Understand.* New York, Ballan-
                         tine, 1990
Winnicott,D.W.   *The Child, the Family, and the Outside World.*
                         Harmondsworth: Penguin, 1964